S0-APP-326

Cosmetic surgery: A consumer's guide

Sylvia Rosenthal

Foreword by Bernard E. Simon, M.D., F.A.C.S.

Tree Communications

J.B. Lippincott Company
Philadelphia and New York

Copyright © 1977 by Tree Communications, Inc.

All rights reserved. First Edition
Printed in the United States of America
2 4 6 8 9 7 5 3 1

Created and produced by Tree Communications, Inc.
250 Park Avenue South, New York, New York

Illustrations by Marina Givotovsky

U.S. Library of Congress Cataloging in Publication Data
Rosenthal, Sylvia Dworsky, birth date
Cosmetic surgery.
Includes index.
1. Surgery, Plastic.   I. Title.
RD119.R68   617'.95   76-58921
ISBN 0-397-01211-X

for Anne, Judy, and Michael

Acknowledgments

Plastic surgery is a demanding, multifaceted specialty that calls upon a wide variety of professional skills and techniques. I have been most fortunate during the preparation of this book in having the advice and critical judgment of many distinguished surgeons and physicians interested in presenting an accurate picture of cosmetic surgery today. They were most generous with their time and knowledge and to all of them I express my heartfelt thanks.

I am deeply grateful:

To Dr. Bernard E. Simon, Dr. Robert Auerbach, Dr. Saul Hoffman, Dr. Peter Linden, and Dr. Victor I. Rosenberg, each of whom took time from their busy professional lives to read portions of the manuscript and to contribute valuable suggestions.

To Dr. Sherrell J. Aston, Dr. Peter Cinelli, Dr. Randolph H. Guthrie, Jr., Dr. Norman Orentreich, Dr. Stanley William Lane, and Dr. Paul S. Striker for their splendid assistance and support.

To Dr. Edgar P. Berry, Dr. Eugene L. Bodian, Mr. Silas A. Braley, Dr. Clayton R. De Haan, Dr. Howard P. Diamond, Dr. John M. Goin, and Dr. Daniel L. Weiner for sharing with me their knowledge and experience.

To Vickie Lindner, my able and dedicated editorial assistant, who contributed three of the chapters, and to Marina Givotovsky, the illustrator.

To Genevieve Young and Nancy Bruning, my editors, whose guidance, vision, and encouragement helped to form this book.

To the scores of women and men who had undergone cosmetic surgery and generously recounted their experiences for these pages.

To the librarians, particularly those at the Jerome P. Webster Library of Plastic Surgery at the College of Physicians and Surgeons, who provided me with a number of authoritative texts.

And to Dr. Theodore Rosenthal for his wise counsel, patience, and unfailing good humor during the period of gestation of this volume.

Sylvia Rosenthal

Contents

Foreword

Since the first humanoid saw its reflection in a forest pool and recognized it for what it was, man (and woman) has been deeply involved with his appearance. The human face and body were immortalized in sculpture by the Ancient Greeks, whose sense of beauty and feeling for proportion has been equaled but never surpassed. It is not surprising that the art and science of medicine arose in this same humanistic tradition. Plastic surgery is the legitimate child of the marriage between concern for form and appearance on the one hand and the art and science of medicine on the other. They are equally important—the plastic surgeon who does not understand basic anatomy, physiology and pathology, the reaction of the tissues to injury and diseases, and the vagaries of wound healing cannot be trusted to perform safely. Similarly, the surgeon without an aesthetic sense and an eye for beauty and proportion is also incapable of producing the best possible results.

To obtain the proper background, today's surgeon must spend a long apprenticeship in basic surgical studies before he commences a rigorous two-to-three-year term of special training in plastic surgery. Indeed, even after entering practice, the dedicated surgeon never stops studying, learning, attending conferences, and sharpening his skills, for he knows that his greatest satisfactions come through professional growth.

The author of this volume is a highly capable writer and researcher who has approached her task with humility and devotion and, indeed, without preconceived notions. She has tempered her enthusiasm for the subject with cold facts and common sense, and has rejected the "miracles-of-plastic-surgery" approach. Nor does she equate plastic surgery with the visit to the beauty parlor—or as one slick magazine entitled it – "The Lunch Hour Lift."

Her information was obtained by spending long hours with a number of my colleagues, all of them distinguished and knowledgeable. They all spent long years studying their craft and perfecting their skills and learning not only when and how to operate but, just as important, when not to!

The author guides the reader through the intricacies of the subject, avoiding the inaccuracies and exaggerations that have characterized so much of what has been written in the popular press.

Plastic surgery is "happy surgery." The closure of a wide cleft of the lip and palate in an infant, relief from the weight of huge, burdensome breasts, the reduction to an attractive size of a grotesquely large nose in an adolescent, the reconstruction of a breast after removal for cancer, the smoothing of a sagging, aged face are all designed to improve self-image and to enhance the enjoyment of life.

However, the "consumer" must remember that this is serious surgery with potential for harm and even disaster. Even in the best hands, good results can be predicted but not guaranteed. So choose your surgeon with the greatest of care. The consumer has every right to ask his surgeon about his training, experience and his hospital and/or medical school affiliations. He should consult his own general practitioner or internist for advice and recommendations. The local County Medical Society or a fine community or teaching hospital will assist in finding a properly trained surgeon. Lastly, there are several national plastic surgery societies who will give you the name of qualified surgeons in your locality.

Bernard E. Simon, M.D., F.A.C.S.
Attending Surgeon and Chief
Division of Plastic Surgery
The Mount Sinai Hospital

1

The Facts about Cosmetic Surgery

Probably no specialty in medicine has been as surrounded by myth and misconception as cosmetic surgery—that branch of plastic surgery concerned with improving the appearance of the face and body, as differentiated from reconstructive surgery in which the aim is to restore congenital or traumatic defects to normal.

Cosmetic or aesthetic surgery (the two terms are interchangeable) is viewed by some patients with what one plastic surgeon ruefully calls the "magical thinking" syndrome. For those persons imbued with magical thinking, aesthetic surgery is the means by which a patient becomes transformed. Whatever defects had been troubling them—a sagging face, wrinkled eyelids, a misshapen nose, breasts that are too large or too small—can be corrected with little or no pain, no convalescent period, no scars, and no complications. In the unreal world of magical thinking, aesthetic surgery is not subject to any of the pitfalls of general surgery and the patients emerge, restored and beautiful—or perhaps handsome—with their problems solved and their frustrations ended.

Other persons, troubled and unhappy over a cosmetic defect, are either unaware that a surgical correction is possible, or fearful of what correction entails and are uncertain of how to go about finding out.

It is the purpose of this book to dispel the myths and fill in the blanks with accurate, specific information about what aesthetic surgery can accomplish on the face, body, skin, and scalp. What *are* its benefits, its risks, its limitations, and its complications? What price must patients be prepared to pay in terms of irreversible body and skin changes, scarring, pain and discomfort, dollars, and time away from their usual activities? Who should have cosmetic surgery? What patients are too old or too young?

To find the answers to these questions, scores of physicians—primarily plastic surgeons, but also oral surgeons, general surgeons, dermatologists, and psychiatrists—and patients were interviewed. The recommendations, opinions, and conclusions of the medical men and the experiences and reactions of the patients are recorded in these chapters. You may notice that, throughout the book, the patients' voices are almost unanimously happy ones. Some patients have reservations about the results but none express regret that the surgery was undertaken. This chorus of approval was not deliberately sought.

About 95 percent of the patients interviewed were referred, not by their surgeons, but by friends of friends. No attempt has been made to select those who would express satisfaction with the results. Rather, it was hoped that a broad range of reactions from good to negative would be encountered, but this did not happen. That is not to say there were no bad results or unhappy patients, because human tissue can be capricious and unpredictable, and the most skilled and experienced surgeons all have case histories in their files they would rather forget about. The most likely conclusion is that there *are* more satisfied patients than dissatisfied ones, and the latter prefer not to talk.

Reconstructive surgery was always considered respectable, but cosmetic surgery, with its emphasis on beauty rather than on function, was thought of as frivolous and slightly outside the realm of serious medicine. It was sought mainly by the rich and by movie stars and people in the theater whose professional survival depended on their keeping their youth and beauty. The operations were performed furtively and patients were secretive and silent.

This has changed. Aesthetic surgery has recently come into its own and gained acceptance. Operations to correct a mistake of nature or to erase some of the signs of aging are now as acceptable as coloring your hair, wearing a wig, or having your teeth capped. Men and women in moderate financial circumstances, willing to make sacrifices to afford the costly operations, are among those filling the waiting rooms of plastic surgeons today. In 1946, according to the American Medical Association, about 15,000 Americans underwent surgery to enhance their appearance. In 1972, this number went up to about 1,000,000 and it is estimated that within the next few years, it will reach 1,500,000. There is little doubt that aesthetic surgery will continue to grow in popularity and that as today's young men and women wrinkle and age, cosmetic operations will be undertaken with less hesitancy than in the previous generation.

It is not difficult to understand the reasons for this boom. To begin with, improved anesthetics and surgical techniques have made it possible for the well-trained plastic surgeon to perform complex and delicate operations safely. The art of aesthetic surgery, honed and refined by the experiences and mistakes of the past, has reached a plateau of excellence. The pinched nose tip or the tight masklike face that proclaimed the hand of the not-so-skillful surgeon is rarely seen these days. Antibiotics have lessened the danger of infection; safe and improved materials for implants have simplified such procedures as increasing the size of chins and breasts, building up noses, and repairing and restoring ears. And even though scars are inevitable when the skin is cut (for that is how nature heals itself), the aesthetic surgeon knows how to hide his tracks. Nose operations, for example, are performed from inside the nostrils as much as possible so the scars are out of sight. Ears, breasts, eyes, and chin have skin folds where a tidy scar can be hidden.

Nevertheless, the surge of interest in self-improvement has not been stimulated only by improved techniques and superior surgical results. It has been nourished by the radio, TV, newspapers, and periodicals which encourage the public to "Pamper your body and soothe your soul." A high value is placed on youth in today's competitive business and social worlds. More and more men, heartened by the examples of prominent figures, are turning to cosmetic surgery. Instead of feeling embarrassed by cosmetic surgery, both men and women are discussing it openly.

We are told, on the other hand, in a number of serious and slightly pejorative studies written by experts in various fields of human behavior, that we are not only a youth-oriented society but a self-oriented one, narcissistic and self-absorbed. Is this a reaction to the Puritan ethic that decreed that vanity was shameful and even wicked? Is it neurotic or is it psychologically healthy to want to look your best, to be good to yourself? Those thousands of well-adjusted persons given an extra measure of self-confidence by cosmetic surgery would have no difficulty answering that last question.

Certainly there is nothing new in the desire to look better or different. Archeological writings and discoveries dating back thousands of years will attest to this. The ancient Assyrians used ivory implants to try to create a strong hooked nose. Chinese women bound their feet to make them dainty. Primitive peoples scarred and distorted their faces and bodies to conform to the prevailing criteria of beauty in their tribe. Influenced by the contemporary concept of what is desirable, personal enhancement has engaged the interest of both sexes throughout history. Styles have changed, but the instinct for personal attractiveness of one kind or another has always existed. Within this century in America, we have had a succession of styles and trends—the buxom Gibson girl, the glamorous, full-bosomed and slightly unreal Hollywood movie star, the flat-chested, short-haired flapper, the all-American girl athlete, and now the abiding interest in preserving the look of youth.

Concepts of beauty are as mercurial as skirt lengths and hair styles, as we can see in the recent shift among young people as to what is beautiful. Only a few years ago, a prominent West Coast plastic surgeon observed that it was almost a ritual for girls whose noses were less than perfect to have their noses remodeled during the summer between high school and college. The operation became a standard high school graduation present. Then came the informal natural look—loose and flowing hair, jeans, T-shirts, and sneakers—and the popularity of movie stars such as Barbra Streisand and Dustin Hoffman, whose faces are very different from the stereotyped perfection that used to fill movie magazines. Noses with bumps ceased to be a matter of concern to young people. The average patient for nasal correction is now in her late twenties or early thirties, married, with children, and a husband who is on his way up the economic scale.

Aesthetic surgery has become part of the mores of late 20th-Century life, not only in America but all over the world. How successful it is and how much it enriches the lives of the persons who seek it depends on a combination of the patients' motivations and expectations, the competence of the surgeon, and, always, the element of luck that protects the patient against unpredictable complications. No guarantee of a perfect or even a good result can be given in any branch of medicine, but the more thorough the surgeon's training, skill, and experience, the greater the chances of a satisfactory result.

How to Find a
Plastic Surgeon

Finding a properly qualified plastic surgeon is the first step toward achieving a good result. It is not a referral you pick up from a newspaper advertisement or a casual mention by your hairdresser. If you know someone who has had a good result from a cosmetic operation similar to one you are interested in, you might ask for the name of the surgeon. This could be a start, but there are many other sources. You can ask your family physician or some other medical specialist you know and trust for names of qualified plastic surgeons.

Other sources are your local County Medical Association and any large teaching or community hospitals in your area. You may write to The American Society of Plastic and Reconstructive Surgeons, Inc., 29 East Madison Street, Suite 807, Chicago, Illinois 60602. All three of these sources will provide the names of reputable plastic surgeons.

You might also consult Marquis' *Directory of Medical Specialists,* available in most large public libraries. This lists physicians according to specialties, and gives their credentials. In the plastic-surgery section, the letters D-PS after the doctors' names stand for *diplomate in plastic surgery,* which means that the physician has been certified by the American Board of Plastic Surgery. In the dental profession, oral surgeons who meet the requirements are certified as diplomates of the American Board of Oral Surgery. Specialists in Canada are certified by the Royal College of Physicians and Surgeons of Canada. To earn this certification, individuals must complete medical school and take a five- to seven-year postgraduate course, which includes thorough training in general surgery and a minimum of two to three years in an approved plastic-surgery training center. They must also take a rigorous written and oral examination that, it might be noted, not everyone passes. Those who fail, naturally, are not certified.

Other specialists who have had specific training in plastic surgery are qualified to perform aesthetic surgery in their fields. Ear, nose, and throat specialists (otolaryngologists) perform corrections of the nose (rhinoplasties) and eye specialists (ophthalmologists) perform cosmetic eyelid surgery. Dermatologists with special training in cosmetic dermatology perform skin planing, chemical peeling, and hair transplants. Your county medical society is a source for these referrals.

An anomalous medical situation exists in this country. As long as physicians are duly licensed in the state in which they are practicing, there is no law that prevents them from performing any medical or surgical procedure they wish, regardless of their competence and training. There is a measure of control by professional organizations and first-rate hospitals which, within their jurisdiction, can prevent inadequately trained physicians from practicing beyond their abilities. But cosmetic surgery is a lucrative field and attracts greedy, incompetent, and unscrupulous physicians who have found ways of circumventing controls. They have established clinics and surgical facilities where there is no supervision except their own. It is hoped that in time the public can be educated to recognize the difference between ethical practitioners who are well trained and qualified and those who operate on the fringes of legitimate medicine, protected by their medical licenses. It should be kept in mind that no ethical board-certified plastic surgeon ever advertises or is associated with any organization that advertises and acts as a referral agency. And that ethical surgeons welcome questions from their patients about their qualifications and training and patients should feel no hesitancy about asking.

The public should be wary of trusting lay operators, regardless of extravagant claims for reviving sagging faces and tired skins. Nothing bad is likely to happen as long as they confine themselves to using bland creams and the gentle laying on of hands, but untold damage has been done when they have moved into chemical and surgical procedures totally beyond their competence. No magic formulas exist that can melt away the signs of aging and there is no substitute for training and knowledge.

The interrelationship of mind and body is present in all illnesses. A feeling of mutual trust between doctor and patient can be most supportive and comforting to the patient recovering from the trauma of aesthetic surgery because it is often an emotionally charged experience. Before committing oneself to a surgeon, it is a good idea to "shop" a bit. Arrange consultations with two or three plastic surgeons. The consultation fees will be well spent and you will have a frame of reference for your final choice. It is desirable that surgeon and patient feel comfortable with each other. One patient reported that she had made up her mind she would take as much time and trouble selecting her surgeon as she had taken shopping for her new car. It was more difficult, because automobile manufacturers advertise and ethical plastic surgeons do not, but she felt she was well rewarded for her efforts.

Patient Selection

The well-adjusted personalities who come to the plastic surgeon with an obvious cosmetic problem that they wish corrected because they'd like to look better present no dilemma to the surgeon. From experience, surgeons know that, barring an unexpected complication, these patients will end up with satisfactory results and be happy patients—which, after all, is what aesthetic surgery is all about.

Aesthetic surgeons also know from experience that in their specialty they deal as often with tangled human emotions as they do with cosmetic defects. The ideal plastic surgeon must be a physician, a surgeon, an artist, and a psychologist. The physician understands the physical condition of the patient and which procedures can be undertaken without endangering the patient's health; the surgeon is equipped with the skills and techniques to achieve a good result; the artist furnishes the aesthetic sense that brings balance and harmony to the corrective surgery; and the psychologist evaluates the patient's aims and expectations in terms of whether they are realistic and possible to achieve. The psychological aspect often presents the greatest challenge to the plastic surgeon at the initial consultation.

Every plastic surgeon knows the frustration of dealing with emotionally unstable or chronically dissatisfied patients who, regardless of the excellence of the results of an operation, can make life difficult for everyone around them, including the surgeon. Sometimes a deep-seated neurosis is at the basis of the patients' unhappiness with their appearance. Unfortunately there is no clear line between the patient who may be helped to solve an inner problem by a change in external appearance and those in whom surgery could precipitate an emotional crisis. Plastic surgeons are understandably reluctant to accept patients who might benefit more from psychiatric counseling than from cosmetic surgery. They often request a psychiatric consultation for patients they are uneasy about, but many depend on their intuition and experience in screening out patients they feel will become postoperative problems.

Certain patterns of behavior act as a warning signal to the experienced plastic surgeon. The patient with a pathological concern out of proportion to the extent of the defect must be carefully evaluated. A good result can be achieved with a pronounced deformity, whereas a slight defect may elude correction. Another warning bell rings when the aesthetic surgeon feels he is unable to communicate or establish a good emotional contact with the patient. Then there are the patients who are unable to state accurately or succinctly what it is about their faces or bodies that displeases them. Their self-image—how they perceive themselves—may be so removed from reality that no alteration of a body part could bring any satisfaction. If a patient with a misshapen nose and excessively wrinkled eyelids is concerned about a minor imperfection such as earlobes that don't quite match, the surgeon is given a clue as to the trouble that lies ahead if surgery is undertaken. A realistic self-image and realistic expectations are the basis of successful aesthetic surgery.

Some patients fix their attention on a defect of a body part—a facial feature or a body contour—on which they blame all their failures. After surgery has failed to provide the expected life changes, the patient's hostility is directed toward the surgeon who becomes the cause of subsequent failures. One plastic surgeon told of a young woman who was extremely distressed over her bulging thighs, which she felt were responsible for the waning interest of her lover. With some reluctance, the surgeon agreed to operate. It was a decision he long regretted because when the relationship between the couple ended, the young woman blamed the surgeon in a series of bitter, acrimonious harangues. She claimed the scars from the operation were responsible for ending the romance.

The "insatiable patient" is another nightmare for surgeons. General surgeons recognize the neurotic patient who seeks surgery as a solution to emotional conflicts. Such patients are addicted not to the physical effects of the surgery, but to the ritual of the hospital, the operative procedure, and the care and attention lavished on them and their bodies. They make repeated demands for further surgery, and the plastic surgeon who accepts them will have reason to regret it. The truly neurotic patient cannot be satisfied.

There is still another reason for careful screening of patients. Physicians in the United States are haunted by the threat of malpractice suits, a situation practically unknown in most other countries. Plastic surgeons are particularly vulnerable and their malpractice insurance premiums are among the highest in the medical profession. The public is litigation-prone, and what used to be a rare hazard has become an ever-present super-nightmare that harasses every physician and surgeon in the United States.

Aesthetic surgeons are not miracle workers, but they can bring harmony and balance to a face and body by correcting imperfections. They emphasize that no one should have aesthetic surgery to please someone else—a mate, family, or sweetheart. Under such circumstances no one will be pleased. The only valid motivation for elective cosmetic surgery is a deep personal desire for self-improvement. It should be undertaken with the realization that no matter how skilled the aesthetic surgeon is, he cannot create beauty where it did not exist, nor can he reverse the aging process, or assure social, professional, or sexual triumphs. The surgeons will be the first to tell you that they can change features, but they cannot change lives.

Fees, Costs, and Procedures

Surgeons' fees for cosmetic operations vary widely, depending on geographical area, the type and complexity of the operation, the patient's requirements, and the individual surgeon's fees. The fees cited in the following chapters for different operations may not reflect those that exist in your area.

It is customary for fees to be paid in advance, although in some special situations the patient and surgeon may work out some other mutually agreeable arrangement. The practice of prepayment has some advantages for both parties: the surgeon is assured of payment and the patient has the comfort of not being faced with the bill later. It has also been found that when patients pay for the surgery in advance, they are more likely to be satisfied with the results. The patient who pays later is often overly critical and finds complaints as a ploy to avoid paying.

The expenses connected with aesthetic surgery (surgeons' and anesthetists' fees and hospital costs) are not covered by medical insurance unless a medical problem is being corrected as well. In these situations, part of the cost is reimbursed by such programs as Blue Cross and Blue Shield. In a typical major-medical policy, benefits are not provided for cosmetic care unless necessitated by injury. Your surgeon's office staff can advise you on these medical/cosmetic matters.

Other items that may be included in your hospital bill are fees for the use of the operating room and recovery room, and any anesthesia and drugs. Costs of aesthetic surgery are income-tax deductible on the same basis as any other medical expenses.

There are a few other preoperative rituals to be observed. Arrangements must be made for the "before" photographs for the surgeon's records. "After" photographs will be added when healing is complete. The frontal and profile photographs serve a number of purposes. They are frequently studied by the surgeon before the operation and often taken into the operating room. They are also the patient's and the surgeon's best evidence in case of a malpractice suit, an important consideration in our litigious society. Some surgeons take their own photographs and others refer their patients to a professional medical photographer. Medical photographers usually charge from $35 to $50 for the "before" and "after" pictures. Some surgeons ask their patients to sign releases in which the patient agrees to recognize the risks of surgery and promises not to expect the impossible from the operation. These documents are of questionable value in court cases because the suing patient can disclaim knowledge of the contents of the release.

Cosmetic surgery may be available for those who cannot afford full fees. Reduced rates for needy people may be arranged at some institutions such as universities and teaching hospitals, children's hospitals, burn-treatment or cleft-palate centers, or in municipal, county, and state hospitals. Contact any large hospital in your community that has a training program for plastic surgeons, or get in touch with your state's equivalent of vocational rehabilitation or crippled children's services. Medicaid pays for some cosmetic operations for the medically indigent under certain conditions.

Purely cosmetic procedures may be a bit more difficult to arrange than reconstructive procedures of injuries, burns, head and neck cancer, or treatment of congenital defects. For further information, you may write to The American Society of Plastic and Reconstructive Surgeons, Inc., mentioned on page 12 in this chapter.

In some parts of the United States there is a growing trend toward performing the cosmetic operations under local anesthesia in the physician's office or in an ambulatory surgical facility. This has come about as a way of coping with the skyrocketing costs of hospitalization. In some large hospitals, an overnight stay has been known to cost up to $1,000. Operations such as face lifts, eyelid corrections, chin implants, and breast augmentations are being performed as outpatient procedures. After surgery, patients are given drugs that reverse the effect of the anesthesia and they go home an hour or so later. The surgeon is always within call, just as he would be if the patient were in a hospital. This practice might have been unthinkable 10 or 15 years ago, but in the last five or six years it has gained wide acceptance and both surgeons and patients express satisfaction with it.

Since most aesthetic surgery is on the head and neck, a large portion of this book deals with correction of defects in these areas; however, coverage has also been given to contour corrections of body defects, from breasts to buttocks. Not all plastic surgeons are in accord about the practicability of some body surgery, and their reservations are noted in the text.

No one who researches the contemporary medical literature on plastic surgery can fail to be impressed by the dedication and competence of today's specialists in this field. The skills of the well-trained American plastic surgeons are not surpassed anywhere else in the world, yet they are constantly striving for better techniques and more perfect results. For the patient undergoing aesthetic surgery, there can be a long interlude between the initial incision and the final visible results, and this interlude is explored in the chapters that follow.

2

The Face Lift

While there are many women and men who take pride in the facial wrinkles and pouches that reflect their earthly experiences, there is a much larger number of those who resent the imprints that time etches on their faces and necks and wish to do something about it. Their motivation transcends vanity, for in view of the premium placed on youth in today's competitive world, it can no longer be considered frivolous for men and women to want to look as good as they can for as long as they can. What else but this universal interest in preserving a youthful, attractive appearance could have propelled the cosmetic business into a multibillion-dollar industry? Certainly Ponce de Leon was never less alone in his quest than he is today.

But in spite of the endless array of creams, lotions, skin tighteners, skin toners, skin fresheners, and other skin-glorifying products that are bought and assiduously used, faces do inevitably show their age. They are not like masks that can be refinished and repainted indefinitely. Some of these commercial products do have value in lubricating and moisturizing the skin and concealing minor irregularities, but those are the limits of their effectiveness.

The inexorable process of aging produces loose, sagging skin, jowls, creases, and wrinkles. Time robs the skin of its elasticity and there is no mechanical gadget or product yet known to science, or even the cosmetic industry, that will make it firm again. As the years pass, the skin stretches and sags and becomes several sizes too big for the face it covers. And with life expectancy of the American people constantly increasing, there is no doubt but that there will be more and more size-12 faces wearing size-16 skins in the future.

The "nonsurgical procedures" that promise to restore a sagging face are a waste of time and money, as anyone who has ever been seduced by the advertisements with their pie-in-the-sky promises will admit. The only way baggy skins can be made to fit the faces and necks once again is by a surgical procedure called a face lift performed by a highly trained plastic surgeon. The face lift is known technically by a number of names: rhytidoplasty (*rhytid* is a Greek word meaning wrinkle); rhytidectomy (the suffix, *ektomē* means excision); and meloplasty, which means plastic surgery of the cheek. But none of these terms quite describes the face lift. It does not excise wrinkles and it goes beyond shaping the cheek. To oversimplify a complex, painstaking procedure, the surgeon incises and detaches the skin of the face and neck, lifts and tightens tissues and muscles underneath it, and shifts and rotates the released skin. The excess skin is trimmed off and the incisions are carefully closed.

A face lift is not a minor undertaking, involving as it does a major dissection of the skin. Actually there is no such thing as a minor operation in plastic surgery. A face lift may not be as critical as a kidney transplant, but it is a procedure that requires an aseptic operating-room setting, some type of anesthesia, usually a hospital stay, and a mandatory period of convalescence of varying lengths during which specific rules must be observed. And as with any other operation, complications can occur.

Surgery such as that performed on the nose, ear, or jaw that involves the framework of the face may be more complex, but the rhytidoplasty is a great challenge to the surgeon. For in this procedure, the surgeon is called upon not to change structure nor to create a new face, but to restore it to a degree of its former youthful symmetry. The surgeon's success in this operation may depend as much on what he does not do as on what he does.

A network of fantasies and distortions has grown around the face lift operation, spurred on in part by the highly publicized stories of women and men who, even before they had their faces lifted, had achieved success through a combination of good looks and talent. And from these glamorous and dramatic results developed the mystique of the face lift. In the minds of many people, the nature, purpose and virtues of the operation have become blurred in a maze of wishful thinking and unrealistic objectives. It is not for people who view it as a solution to major problems in their lives.

One eminent plastic surgeon had this to say: "Hollywood and television and glossy-paper high-fashion magazines have glamorized the face lift to such a degree that people's expectations far surpass what can be reasonably expected. The best results are for people who want to change their appearance for their own benefit. Those who have the surgery to please others may be in for a disappointment. A woman's face lift will probably not bring her wandering husband home or light up a dying romance. It could conceivably help a middle-aged actor portray a younger character in a play or even in a television commercial, but it is highly unlikely that it will help his brother get elected president of the board of his company. It is something that

21

should be considered only for the right reasons—mainly, a more pleasing self-image."

The Face Lift Comes of Age

No one knows exactly who performed the first face lift, but it seems quite certain that it was being done at the turn of the century by a number of surgeons in Europe and a few in America. While some eminent surgeons showed considerable interest in cosmetic facial surgery in the early 1900s, little was written about it. Consequently, there is a lack of information available about the early history and development of face lifting.

The main reason for this curtain of secrecy was that the face lift operation was not considered entirely respectable. In the minds of some, it straddled a thin line between ethical medical practice and quackery. It was regarded as a surgical procedure that pandered only to vanity, and vanity in the Victorian era was distinctly sinful.

Many of the leading surgeons in the early part of the 20th Century disapproved heartily of cosmetic surgery. They believed there was no excuse for surgery outside of that which was required to save life, lessen pain, or improve a crippling deformity. They considered cosmetic surgery dangerous, trivial, and a capricious act on the part of both surgeon and patient. It might be noted that this attitude has persisted through the years among some medical men, although it has lessened considerably in recent times. But there are still those who are not convinced, as illustrated by the internist who recently vehemently berated a patient when she asked him to refer her to a plastic surgeon. "Unadulterated vanity," he thundered. "I'll have no part of it."

To avoid the censure of their colleagues, the surgeons in the early part of this century performed their operations as office procedures or in small private hospitals away from the arenas of large hospitals and teaching centers. Working under these conditions often limited the extent of the surgery and the extent of the improvement they could effect. This situation has been paralleled in more recent times when people in important positions in hospitals, universities, and other institutions used their influence to hinder the practice of face lifting. Many eminent plastic surgeons were obliged to take their face lift surgery to private hospitals or to list the operation under a name that was more acceptable to the hospital administration. This hostile climate undoubtedly kept many talented surgeons from refining and developing techniques further.

Among the pioneers in plastic surgery was a Parisian dermatologist, Madame le Docteur Suzanne Noël, who was noted for her minor office surgery. She cut off small pieces of skin in those areas of the face that needed to be lifted and where she

22

could conceal the scars. It was a modest operation with an equally modest result. Another innovator was Dr. Charles Conrad Miller of Chicago. He was probably the first American to publish exclusively on cosmetic surgery. His first paper on the subject appeared in 1907 and his textbook on cosmetic surgery was published 17 years later. It is interesting to note that the basic face lifting operation performed by most surgeons today is essentially the same as Miller's. Not much has been added.

The earliest face lifts were similar to what is today called a mini-lift. Sometimes the operation consisted of the removal of a strip of skin behind the hairline in the temple region of the face. This brought some slight temporary improvement to the wrinkles of the forehead and around the eyes, but did nothing for the lower part of the face. In another type of operation, a strip of excess skin in front of, below, and just behind the ear was excised. There was little or no undermining. Undermining is the procedure in which the surgeon releases or separates the skin from the fat and muscles that lie beneath it. It is a crucial step in the face lift operation, the one that gives the face lift its long-lasting result. The amount of undermining determines whether the operation is extensive, medium, or just a touch-up face lift. Extensive undermining of the face and neck was probably not done until the 1920s.

These early, timid techniques were as ineffective then as they are today and many knowledgeable surgeons are at a loss to account for the resurgence of interest in the mini-lift procedure, except, perhaps for a patient who has had repeated face lifts and is determined to keep ahead of the slightest sag at any cost. One plastic surgeon commented that a mini-lift is a step backward to horse-and-buggy days and kerosene lamps. He observed that a mini-lift gives a mini-result at a maxi-price.

The ineffectiveness of these first baby-step operations and their short-lived improvements spurred innovative and creative plastic surgeons to develop new techniques. Advances in anesthesia helped to minimize risk as well as to encourage more extensive undermining, which results in dramatic improvement. The well-trained modern plastic surgeons, secure in their knowledge of the position of important ear and facial nerves and muscles and of major blood vessels, are able to tighten and re-drape a sagging face with some striking results.

There is some improvement, too, in the willingness to share surgical techniques among the present generation of young plastic surgeons. This is in contrast to surgeons of an earlier generation who, when they developed new techniques, guarded them closely and imparted their secrets to younger colleagues only with the greatest reluctance. In the last 20 to 25 years or so, there has been a somewhat freer exchange of ideas and methods. The plastic surgeons of today recognize the importance of aesthetic surgery in modern life and take pride in their work.

The face lift has finally come out of the shadows and has gained wide acceptance among people of all ages, in all income brackets and social classes. The plastic surgeons are no longer impelled to hide their face lift patients in anonymous little private hospitals or to rename a face lift procedure. The doctors have seen the demand for this surgery rise sharply over the last ten years among both men and women because the results are almost consistently satisfactory.

Men Discover Cosmetic Surgery

It is interesting to note that about 15 to 20 percent or more of the requests for face lifts and eyelid surgery now come from men. This is a change from a time not so long ago when the waiting rooms of cosmetic surgeons were the exclusive domain of women, except for the occasional presence of an anxious husband or father. Although this is not a typical experience, one New York surgeon with a large following in the arts commented that about half of his patients are men. But the lure of the rejuvenation techniques of cosmetic surgery extends to males other than those in the arts. It attracts men from all walks of life—business, politics, finance, sports, law, and other professions, many of whom have no hesitancy in talking freely about their facial surgery. These open discussions are making men less self-conscious about having cosmetic surgery, and, at least in the large cities, fewer quizzical looks are directed at the men who elect to have it.

It has taken almost 70 years, but the face lift operation has finally become socially and medically acceptable.

The Aging Process

Occasionally, one sees men and women in their seventies whose faces are still aglow with a youthful bloom that has somehow managed to elude the passage of time. But they are the exceptions. For most mortals, the process of deterioration wins the race against the ability of the skin and its underlying tissues to avoid showing the patina of age. All soft tissues of the body eventually sag, drawn earthward by the relentless pull of gravity.

The process of aging begins gently, almost imperceptibly, at about 25 or 30. In some cases, it might even start at the end of the teens. Fine superficial lines—usually horizontal—etch the forehead and the area around the eyes. People who have the habit of squinting and wrinkling their brow will speed up and intensify the formation of lines in the areas involved in these facial movements. As people progress into their late thirties and early forties, the subcutaneous fat in the neck begins to shrink.

24

The neck is a common site for the revealing signs of aging. Deep lines often ring it to mark out the years, just as in trees. The loosening of the skin of the neck may also create vertical lines or folds. The nasolabial folds that run downward from the outside rim of the nose to the corners of the mouth deepen; frown lines crease the forehead; and wrinkles begin to appear around the eyes.

Within another decade the skin of the neck has relaxed further and jowls may begin to mar the smooth contour of the chin and jawline. A groove from the angle of the mouth traces an uneven and swirling path along its way to the border of the jaw. Fine lines radiate out above the upper margin of the mouth. It would seem that equality of the sexes does not extend to the ability of both men and women to keep a firm upper lip, for men rarely have these lines—a source of annoyance to their wives. The skin of the male upper lip is not so likely to wrinkle because of its thickness and the layer of connective tissues beneath it, which hold the large and abundant hair follicles. In addition, the abrading action of constant shaving has the effect of tightening and thickening skin, strengthening its resistance to wrinkles.

Around the age of 60, the changes in the skin become deeper lines and grooves, pouches and sags. An unmistakable reminder of the aging process often lies in the eyelids and areas around the eyes. For some people, the crepey saggy eyelids and pouches under the eyes are a familial trait, while in others they mark off the passage of years.

As time goes on, the skin continues to lose its resiliency; more subcutaneous fat is lost and the skin becomes thinner and dryer and more wrinkled. Bone and muscles atrophy. In old age, the corners of the mouth tend to droop, the nose tip falls, and sagging skin behind the ear causes the ear lobes to elongate.

However, this solemn progression of events and changes does not affect everyone at the same time or to the same degree. The telltale marks of aging do not follow a strictly defined timetable. There are many variables that can hasten or delay the signs of aging, heredity among them. The probabilities for long life and youthful appearance—or the opposite—may have been determined by genetic accident long before the person involved was in control. Also affecting the aging process are type of skin, body build, life style, facial habits, and exposure to the elements. It should be noted here that excessive exposure to sunlight is one of the greatest offenders in aging and deterioration of the skin, particularly for people with light complexions.

There is still another factor in the process of aging, but it has nothing to do with years or heredity. It is an individual's emotional response to the traumas and frustrations of life—their reactions to stress. No one can hope to live without stress, but those who learn to cope with it will hold on to the freshness and vitality of youth a little longer. Profound, uncontrolled emotion leaves its imprint on our faces for the world to see.

Candidates for the Face Lift

Some skins and facial structures are better suited to successful rhytidoplasties than others. High on the list of desirables would be people in their late forties or early fifties with a minimum of wrinkles or scars, whose skin hangs in folds, contains little underlying fat, and retains a measure of elasticity. Slender people with soft skins, high cheekbones and nicely defined jaw lines are particularly good candidates.

But this is not always the type of patient who comes seeking a face lift, as the surgeons well know. However, the experienced surgeons know how to take advantage of their techniques to achieve the best possible results on all types of faces and skins.

On the other hand, surgeons do not hesitate to refuse a patient who, for one reason or another, they feel is a poor prospect for face lift surgery. They will explain exactly why they do not recommend the operation. Patients should heed this kind of advice when it comes from an ethical, knowledgeable plastic surgeon. It is entirely proper for them to get another opinion, but if it confirms the previous one, they should try to understand it is their well-being that is being given prime consideration. There have been too many cases of people who were so eager for cosmetic surgery that they rejected sound advice and searched until they found a doctor willing to perform the operation they wanted. Every profession has its share of greedy, self-seeking members. The results of this unrecommended surgery were often disastrous.

Age offers no particular restrictions for people considering face lifts, which, after all, are directed toward slowing up the progression of aging in middle life and rejuvenating the already well-wrinkled segment of the population. It is highly unusual, but there have been isolated instances of a teenage patient or one in the early twenties who, because of a combination of physiological and psychological factors, required a face lift and was considered acceptable. At the other end of the time clock are people in their seventies who may be candidates for cosmetic surgery if they are in good physical and mental health. If their skins have lost elasticity, are leathery in texture, and are heavily crossed with wrinkles and sags, the results of the face lift could be less than satisfactory. Some of the wrinkles and folds could be reduced, but the greatest improvement would be in eliminating the excess facial skin and improving the sagging neck. One plastic surgeon was as delighted as his 74-year-old patient, a former headmistress of a school, with the results of her third face lift.

No broad generalization would cover every case, but probably the ideal age and the one at which one could expect the greatest improvement and the most lasting result would be the late forties and early fifties, when the skin and muscles are still firm and elastic. As might be expected, the majority of face lift patients are in that age group. What impels them to have the surgery?

"I decided to have a face lift because my face looked old and my body didn't," said Arthur P., a slim, dapper 51-year-old businessman. "I just wanted to synchronize them. My face was one big sag and I had one of those turkey-neck throats that got in the way of my collars and ties—and as for wearing a turtleneck sweater—forget it." The beige turtleneck he was wearing was neat and tidy on a neat and tidy neck. "It seemed like a pretty bold undertaking because, while I had heard of men who had had face lifts, I didn't know any. Anyway, I did it and I'm satisfied that my face matches my body and how I feel."

Lenore R. is typical of the chic, perfectly groomed women one sees in exclusive resorts, in expensive shops, and at glossy charity balls. She is 62 and has just had her second face lift, ten years after the first. "I have a devoted, wonderful husband who I'm sure never noticed the sags in my face and neck. I'm not striving for everlasting youth—I know that's impossible, but my standards are high . . . . I like order and beauty. I try to have it in my home, my clothes, in my relationships with people, and I want it in myself. Maybe it's vanity, but if vanity makes us reach out and try a little harder, it can't be such a bad thing."

"I felt it would be advantageous to my career if I looked younger," said Adele G., a 53-year-old divorcée. She is a successful executive in a youth-oriented business. The year before she had the face lift, she went through the disillusioning experience of seeing her husband go off with a woman 20 years her junior. She was shattered physically and emotionally. But an important promotion in her firm made her take stock of herself. "I was appalled at the way I looked," she said. "My face was a mass of lines and bags. I looked old and tired ... some image for an executive in a firm whose work revolves around the interests of children and young people. I was looking years removed from the age group I was supposed to be responsive to. I knew I had to do something to help myself."

Noncandidates for the Face Lift

Age may not necessarily deter anyone from considering a face lift operation, but the patient's physical condition might. Anyone who is not in good health or who is suffering from a chronic disease that would affect healing ability is well advised to postpone planning for the surgery until the condition improves and

27

the internist gives permission. And no one in the midst of an emotional crisis should entertain any thought of cosmetic surgery until their situation stabilizes or they reach the point where they feel they can cope with their problems and look forward.

Postponement of surgery is advised for people who are planning to lose weight. Certainly a prospective candidate for a face lift should delay plans for surgery until he or she has reached the desired weight-loss goal. As anyone who has ever lost a considerable amount of weight knows, the face sags as the pounds melt away. Scarcely a worthwhile prospect for the expensive and hard-won rhytidoplasty. A slight—with emphasis on the slight—gain in weight could enhance the appearance of the face, but the patient must scrupulously avoid an excessive weight gain. A Ping-Pong pattern of fluctuating weight is undesirable for anyone, but in the case of people who have had face lifts, the recurrent stretching of the skin can be disastrous. However, it seems logical to assume that those people who cared enough about how they looked to seek plastic surgery in the first place would also be sufficiently vain and enough interested to keep an unwavering eye on their calorie count and on the indicator on their bathroom scale.

Surgeons are always cautious about advising facial surgery for people whose skins have a tendency to heal with heavy scars such as keloids or hypertrophic scars. This tendency may be present in all types of skins but it is more apt to occur in black skins. With this in mind, surgeons examine candidates for cosmetic surgery carefully to look at old scars which reveal the patient's healing pattern. Keloids are an overgrowth of normal scar tissue. They are usually wider, firmer, and thicker than normal scars. They may remain raised during the patient's lifetime or even grow larger over the years. Not all heavy scars are keloids, although frequently the hypertrophic scar is mistakenly called a keloid. The hypertrophic scar grows larger during the first few months after surgery or an injury, but unlike the true keloid, it slowly softens over the following months. Treatment of the true keloid is difficult and the outcome is uncertain. Sometimes x-ray treatment and injections of cortisone are used, but the results are unpredictable.

The predisposition toward keloids does not necessarily mean that they will develop in face lift scars following surgery. However, it is not unusual for the scars behind the ears to become thickened or hypertrophic, and anyone who has this tendency, black people in particular, must be made aware of this possibility. On the other hand, black skin is less subject to conspicuous wrinkling as it ages.

No one ever makes the decision to have a face rehabilitation on the spur of the moment. The segment of the population old enough to consider the operation is well past the first flush of youth when impetuous actions take precedence over carefully thought out plans. It is important for people contemplating a face lift to understand what it can and cannot do.

What the Prospective Face Lift Patient Should Know

A face lift does not have the power to create beauty. It is a repair job, not a magical means to achieve personal perfection. Bone and cartilage structures are left unchanged, so the operation can restore only a measure of the beauty that once existed, if indeed it ever did. Unlike surgery of the nose, chin, or jaw, it cannot alter a gross physical defect of the bony framework of the face. It cannot create symmetry in a face that lacks it. Nor can it change an oily, large-pored skin into a creamy confection.

It can correct conditions such as generalized sagging of the face and neck, a jowly jaw line, and wattles—the loose, sagging flesh under the chin that forms a cord along the length of the neck. In some cases, it may bring some slight improvement to the brow and eyelids. The lifting and tightening of the facial skin and neck creates a more youthful appearance that generally brings with it a feeling of self-confidence and the psychological lift that is experienced by people who like the way they look.

There are a number of conditions that require additional measures and it would be the exceptional person, who, in later life, did not need more than a single procedure to rejuvenate an aging face. The face lift cannot remove excess crepey skin and bags around the eyes. This correction requires an operation called blepharoplasty (Chapter 3), a name that will come as no surprise to a student of Greek, since *blepharon* means eyelid in that language. The presence of a pronounced double chin may call for another surgical procedure called a submental lipectomy, in which the fat pad just beneath and behind the chin is removed. This procedure is discussed later in this chapter.

Below are other conditions for which the standard face lift is ineffective, and the methods recommended to alleviate them.

Horizontal lines in forehead. These deep furrows present a difficult problem. Treating them surgically is not justified by the result. Sometimes they respond to chemical peeling (Chapter 7). Results last an average of two years, but to maintain the result, the patients would need to retrain themselves not to wrinkle their brow excessively.

Vertical lines between eyebrows. Surgery for these lines is not successful. Some doctors recommend liquid-silicone injections (Chapter 7) but there is a considerable difference of opinion over its use.

29

Nasolabial folds (lines from nose to mouth). This is one of the most disappointing aspects in the present-day face lift techniques. The most one can expect from a face lift is a slight softening of these lines. Patients are frequently frustrated and unhappy after a face lift when the nasolabial folds have not been greatly improved. Cutting out the fold of skin would create a scar. Sometimes silicone injections are recommended by the doctors who approve their use.

Fine, dry wrinkles (sometimes called "prune skin"). These may be treated by either surgical skin planing (dermabrasion) or chemical peeling (Chapter 7), depending upon the patient's type of skin. The results range from indifferent to excellent. When the results are good, they may last for years, but this, too, varies with the individual.

Fine vertical wrinkles that furrow the upper lip. Chemical peeling can be successful in selected cases. Results usually last for several years, but the length of time may vary.

Self-inflicted wrinkles. Mention should be made of the facial habits that are responsible for many of the lines that etch people's faces. People who are in the habit of making broad exaggerated facial movements such as grimacing, squinting, or otherwise distorting their faces will have more and deeper lines than those whose facial expressions are habitually more tranquil. The reason is simple. The skin of the face is unique in that it has many sets of tiny muscles that are attached directly to it, in contrast to the rest of the body, in which the muscles are attached to the bones. These facial muscles control skin movements and make possible the subtle fleeting expressions that sweep across the face with hints of joy, elation, surprise, or anger, pain, or doubt—reactions that reflect with the most delicate precision what the person is thinking and feeling. Without these muscles, faces would be as impassive as a Halloween mask—and as interesting to watch as a bowl of oatmeal.

But the face pays a penalty for being able to show these fine shades of feeling. When muscles are attached to bones as they are everywhere else in the body, wrinkles do not form. The muscles of the face, however, contract when they are called into play to express an emotion. With the contractions, a series of furrows are created in the skin. As the skin loses its resiliency, the furrows become deeper and eventually take on permanency as lines and wrinkles. People who never frown would not be likely to develop the deep, vertical lines between the eyebrows that are so unwelcome. Patients who continue to wrinkle their brow after the horizontal lines on their forehead are treated and removed are courting the return of the lines.

The universal question from patients contemplating a face lift is how long it will last. It is difficult for a doctor to predict with certainty the exact duration of a face lift, since there are so many variables that may affect the outcome. Face lifts done on people in their forties may last longer than those performed on people in their late fifties and sixties because the younger skin has more elasticity and may not sag as quickly. How old the patient was when the face lift was done, the patient's physical and mental health, the type of skin and the degree of elasticity, the patient's ability to maintain stable weight, and the patient's life style all have an influence on its duration. If the doctor is aware of a specific condition that will affect the lasting quality of the face lift, he (or she) will so inform the patient. Usually the improvement from a properly executed face lift will last from five to ten years or even longer. The improvement brought about by the face lift will gradually diminish over the entire period; there is no possibility of the face *suddenly* reverting to its previous state.

Patients must understand that while the face lift will make them look younger, it cannot stop the biological clock from ticking. Though patients with successful face lifts may look 35 when they are 45, they will not look 35 forever. The aging process will take place on the "new" face as it did on the old, and gradually patients will appear older, although they will probably look somewhat younger and better than they would have without the operation.

Evelyn B., a brisk, peppy 56-year-old who has a healthy, realistic view of her situation, says:

Certainly I have lines and droops in my face that weren't there five years ago when I had my face lift operation, but when I look at my contemporaries, I still feel I'm ahead. My doctor gave me no guarantee that this wouldn't happen so I'm not disappointed.

Evelyn's comment about the "no guarantee" applies to every branch of medicine. There are no doctors or surgeons, however well trained and skillful, who can give a patient complete assurance of a perfect or even a good result in every case. Healing of tissue is affected by several factors, some of which are beyond the control of the surgeons. Medicine is not an exact science and results can be unpredictable. But the more thorough the surgeon's training and experience, the greater the chances for a satisfactory result.

It should be clearly understood that all surgery that begins with an incision must end with a scar. But with concealment of scars high on the priority list of plastic surgeons, they make the inci-

Duration of Face Lift

Face Lift Scars

sions for the face lift in areas covered by hair, in the natural fold of the skin directly in front of the ear, and in areas not normally exposed to view, as behind the ear. As a result, the scarring from a well-executed face lift is minimal. The fine hairline scar in front of the ear can scarcely be seen after a few months when healing is complete, and judicious makeup can make it invisible. Although the majority of people do not have more than one or two face lifts in a lifetime, there is no limit to the number that may be performed if the patient is in good health. The new incisions are placed so that they eliminate the scar tissue from previous face lifts and there are no additional scars.

The Consultation   Many prospective patients come to their first meeting with the plastic surgeon feeling tense and anxious. Most likely they have done a good deal of soul-searching about whether or not to have the surgery. They may have had to wrestle with their conscience to justify wanting an operation that, unlike other kinds of necessary and life-saving surgery, is elective and not a crisis situation. They may be fearful of pain and discomfort and concerned over ultimate results. For many, the operation represents a sacrifice in time and money, particularly the latter, and they may feel guilty about the expenditure. But in spite of all this, the patient comes hoping to hear that an operation is indicated. It is ironic that the usual wish for a verdict of "no surgery" is reversed when it is a plastic surgeon who is being consulted.

The first consultation may take anywhere from 15 minutes to half an hour or more. It is a time for mutual appraisal between surgeon and patient. The surgeon must decide whether the patient's expectations are realistic and whether the operation requested can yield significant results that will last a reasonable length of time. Lovely young women who plaintively point out lines and shadows that can scarcely be seen, people whose faces have structural defects that no amount of skin shifting can improve, and the emotionally unstable are not unknown to plastic surgeons.

On the other side of the desk is the patient gathering impressions that will build a relationship of confidence—or lack of it—that has nothing to do with the ability of the surgeon. Knowing other patients who were successfully treated by the surgeon can help establish a climate of trust. But if patients do not feel this trust and confidence and seem unable to establish a rapport with the surgeon, they should seek another doctor.

The surgeons base their decisions on whether the patient is a good candidate for surgery by questioning the patient and evaluating the physical condition. Adele G., who has been quoted earlier, describes what happened:

The doctor asked me a lot of questions—what bothered me most; why I wanted the operation; what did I expect to happen as a result. I was very frank—I told him about the breakup of my marriage and how it affected me. I told him about my new job and why it was important for me to look my best. And I told him that mostly I was weary of the bags and sags and lines and wrinkles in my face. I assured him that I had no notion that having my face lifted would bring a knight in shining armor to my doorstep. All I wanted was my own face back, but a younger version.

The surgeon studies each area of the prospective patient's face. Is the excess skin in the lower lid a defect of the lid or is it part of the sagging of the adjacent cheek? If the latter, the face lift alone might take care of it without eyelid repair. What about the chin line? Will the face lift make it tidy or will further correction be needed? The surgeon must also satisfy himself that the patient is in good enough physical condition to meet the stress of anesthesia, surgery, and rehabilitation. The surgeon will also seek out any hidden condition that might be affected by the intended operation. He must know whether the patient heals well or with certain types of scars. He must be concerned with whether the patient is suffering from any systemic disease, hypertension, and/or any bleeding or blood clotting disorder that would require treatment in advance of surgery. If he has any doubts about the patient's physical condition, he may ask for a medical opinion from the patient's doctor.

If the surgeon feels that the patient's motivations for and expectations of the surgery are sound, he will recommend what he thinks should be done. Adele was pleased with what the doctor had to say.

I'd been worried that I'd be sent home with a pat on my back and the sags in my face, but instead the doctor said I needed an entire face rehabilitation—a face lift, eyelid surgery, and a chemical peel on my upper lip and chin. He explained that the face lift would not do anything for the fine wrinkles on my upper lip that my lipstick was always running into, and the chemical peel was the best way to get rid of them. He would do all three procedures at the same operation.

But he certainly didn't make me any promises. He said he couldn't make me beautiful if I wasn't beautiful before, or give me high cheekbones if I didn't have them. He said I'd still be myself but I'd look better and fresher and that when I went back to work, no one would have any trouble recognizing me—which was exactly what I wanted.

The surgeon explains what each procedure means in terms of discomfort, time needed for convalescence, and possible complications. At this time, the patient should ask questions about anything that is troubling or puzzling, for this may be the only meeting the patient will have with the surgeon before the operation. A word from Adele:

The doctor went into great detail about the operation and what he was going to do and why—and I asked a lot of questions, but I should have been told more about what happens after the operation. For instance, if I had been told why my eyes might feel tight and teary, and why my face would feel numb, and understood that these were usual symptoms ... and that they would be temporary ... I'm sure I wouldn't have been so worried. And I should have been told to have proper makeup at home for when I needed it instead of having to shop for it while my lip and chin were still bright crimson from the chemical peel. I was terribly self-conscious about going into a store. None of this was a serious omission, but having the information in advance would have made me a little more comfortable.

The doctor assumes that all questions were answered during the consultation, but in many cases the information has set off a chain reaction and generated more questions in the patient's mind. The patient should not hesitate to ask the doctor for another appointment before the surgery, if she desires it.

There is always a fee for the consultation, even if the surgeon declines to operate. The surgeon is entitled to a fee, since his knowledge and time were spent on examination and interviewing. However, the prospective patient will not be charged for an additional visit if it is requested. Consultation fees range from $25 to $45, depending on the surgeon.

Before Surgery

If the consultation between surgeon and patient has gone well and each is satisfied with the other, the arrangements for the operation are put into motion. The surgeon's office takes care of the hospital reservations, and the date for the operation is set. The majority of surgeons perform their operations in hospitals although there are a few who maintain operating rooms in their office quarters that are as well equipped, staffed, and as aseptic as those in hospitals.

Details of fees and payment are clarified and the "before" pictures are scheduled. The use of photographs is important to the surgeon in the preoperative planning. Bold and unflattering, these pictures pinpoint the process of aging in the eyes, face, and neck. Many surgeons take them into the operating room and refer to them during the operation.

Doctors may no longer find it necessary to conceal their face lifting operations, but this does not extend to all patients. Most people are perfectly willing to talk about it, but there are still a few who prefer to keep their plans for such surgery a deep, dark secret. They may tell a few close friends but they generally use a variety of ruses to explain their absence from their customary haunts or places of business. A two- or three-week vacation, destination undisclosed, is a popular ploy and gains credibility when the traveler returns looking fresh and rested.

One plastic surgeon, with obvious relish, recounts the strategy used by one of his self-conscious male patients who was determined to keep his face lift operation a private matter. To do this, he created what is known in military circles as a diversionary tactic. Immediately after the operation he grew a moustache so that, when he returned to work two weeks later, the new moustache was the focal point of his face and no one doubted that he had grown it during his vacation in the Canadian Rockies. A couple of months later he shaved it off and all his friends marveled at how much younger he looked without it.

In preparation for the surgery, patients are advised not to take aspirin or any other drug containing salicylates (Bufferin, Anacin, Excedrin, etc.) for two weeks before and after surgery. This is a precautionary measure because aspirin can cause increased bleeding during and following the operation, which may increase the risk of a complication. Medications such as Tylenol and Datril are recommended as substitutes. Women are advised to discontinue any hormone medication for ten days to two weeks before surgery.

Patients are routinely admitted to the hospital the day before surgery. Medical tests are done on urine, blood, heart, lungs, and blood pressure. The night before surgery, the patients wash their faces and necks thoroughly and give themselves a 15-minute shampoo, using an anti-bacterial soap such as pHisoHex. The cleansing action is an additional safeguard against infection. Patients scheduled for general anesthesia are asked not to eat or drink for eight hours before the operation.

Anesthesia

The face lift operation may be done under local or general anesthesia, but the anesthesia of choice for most plastic surgeons is the local with preoperative sedatives, begun at bedtime the night before surgery. By the time the patients are wheeled into the operating room, they are completely relaxed and drowsy. There are a number of reasons for the preference for local anesthesia. For one, it is simpler to control bleeding when a local anesthesia is used in conjunction with epinephrine (Adrenalin). Also, some surgeons prefer to be able to watch the patient's normal expression during surgery, which cannot be done when the patient is completely unconscious under general anesthesia. The local anesthesia does away with the need for the endotracheal tube used in general anesthesia. This is the tube that carries the anesthetic gas through the mouth and into the trachea, or windpipe. It can obscure a portion of the face, and if surgery is planned for the area around the mouth, this could be inconvenient. Patients who have had face lifts and eyelid surgery and other procedures at the same time under local anesthesia report they had no pain or discomfort during the operation. Injections can be repeated if the effects of the anesthesia begin to wear off during the course of the surgery, and sometimes Valium is given intravenously. This is Adele's recollection:

A pill at bedtime and I slept the sleep of the blessed. Another pill in the morning before the operation and half an hour or so later—not that I had any sense of time—another pill. I floated off in a bubble through peach-colored corridors to the operating room ... at least that's how it seemed to me. I remember practically nothing from then on. The operation took about four and a half hours and I'm told I talked with the surgeon during the operation. They tell me I had visitors that night and carried on a coherent conversation with them, but I have no recollection of anything until I woke up the next morning.

However, for the patients who are fearful of being conscious during any kind of surgery, general anesthesia is used. There are some surgeons who prefer it because they feel that patients grow restive during the lengthy face lift, impeding the work and interfering with the concentration of the surgeon. This procedure requires the services of a highly skilled, experienced anesthesiologist.

Local anesthesia is administered by the surgeon. Sometimes a system called local standby is used in which the patient receives local anesthesia attended by an anesthesiologist who monitors the patient throughout the operation. When the surgeon administers the local anesthesia there is no charge. Anesthesiologists' fees start at about $300 and go up to 20 percent of the surgical fee.

The Rhytidoplasty   It should be understood that although the aims of all plastic surgeons are the same—to bring about the greatest possible improvement in the patient's appearance and to have a happy patient—there is no standardization of methods among them. No single account of a surgical procedure or patient management can reflect widespread medical practices, for all surgeons have their techniques and personal maneuvers that work well for them and with which they are comfortable. Some surgeons are more innovative; some more traditional in their methods— there can be many pathways to a satisfactory result. This variety of approach applies to almost every step of the face lifting operation, from pre-operative procedures, through placement of incisions, type of dressings, and removal of stitches, to postoperative care.

The rhytidoplasty usually takes from 2½ to 4 hours, depending on how much is to be done and with what speed the surgeon works. Often the operation is done in conjunction with the eyelid operation, which takes from 1½ to 2 hours. Some surgeons prefer not to combine the two, but to perform them separately when both procedures are indicated. But whether they are done together or separately is a matter for the surgeon and the patient to decide.

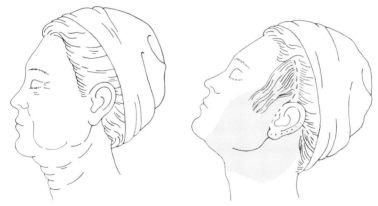

A candidate for a face lift has a sagging face and loose neck. An incision is made (dashed line) and the skin is undermined (shaded area).

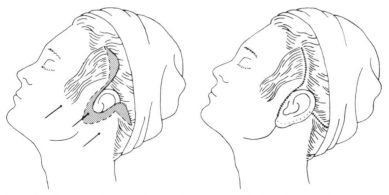

The skin is rotated upward, creating excess skin (shaded area). Excess skin is trimmed and final sutures are made.

The number and location of incisions will vary, depending on whether the patient is a man or a woman, the presence (or absence) of hair, and what the doctor hopes to accomplish. In most cases, the incision is started in the hair-bearing scalp in the region of the temples. The hair has been previously parted, exposing the section of the scalp where the incision is to be made. The incision continues down approximately to the point where the ear is attached to the head. It continues downward to the natural crease immediately in front of the ear, curves around the earlobe, along the back of the ear, and slopes into the neck hairline along a previously prepared strip of scalp. The hair in this pathway is either trimmed or shaved, according to the surgeon's preference. The positioning of this last incision varies according to the hairstyle worn by a man or a woman. Women who wear their hair in an upsweep would need to have the incision placed higher. Surgeons avoid making incisions exactly at the hairline for obvious reasons. In the case of balding men with sufficient hair on their temple regions, the incision might start immediately above the ear within the hair of the temples and continue down, around, and behind the ear, curving back into the hair of the scalp.

A large flap of skin is created from each incision line downward. The surgeon then undermines (separates the skin from the fat and muscle that lie underneath it), starting from the back of the ear and proceeding toward the jaws. The amount of undermining depends on the amount and location of the sagging, drooping skin and it may need to go deep into the neck both in front and behind the ears.

The surgeon proceeds with the undermining, using infinite care not to injure the important facial nerve and its branches, the muscles, and important blood vessels. In the hair-bearing regions such as the temples, the undermining must be done deeply so as not to disturb the hair follicles. Some of the tiny nerve endings in the skin are disturbed during the undermining, causing the feeling of numbness that patients experience following a face lift. In two or three months, when the interrupted nerve endings become rejoined through the natural process of healing, normal sensation will be restored.

Some surgeons shift and tighten the tissues under the skin to provide a firm foundation for the transposed skin, but there is no general agreement among plastic surgeons about the necessity for this step. There is another school of thought that believes that rotating and redraping the undermined skin is sufficient for a good and lasting result without disturbing the subcutaneous tissues.

After the undermining, the surgeon gently rotates and redrapes the skin which is then tailored to fit the face. Anchor sutures are placed above and behind the ear, the excess skin is trimmed, and the incisions are sutured. Generally the incision in front of the ear is the last to be closed. This procedure is then repeated on the other side of the face. The two sides are always done in sequence, not simultaneously, in order to achieve the greatest degree of symmetry between the two halves of the face. Sometimes a small piece of soft rubber tubing is left in the incision to allow drainage of secretions and blood.

In the face lift, the surgeon's primary concern is the skin—how extensive the area is that should be undermined, in which direction it should be rotated and pulled, and how much should be cut away. The critical judgment needed to make these decisions is what makes surgery an art and not just a science. Training, experience, and skill are all brought into play as the surgeon handles the delicate tissues. The greater the area of undermining, the greater the possibility of complications. In addition, if too much skin is removed, the resulting tension can create a frozen expression, or cause broad scarring or a degree of distortion to the eyes, nose, or mouth. The surgeon must attain the right balance between overachieving and the other extreme, for if too little skin is removed, the æsthetic improvement may be minimal and the patient will be disappointed in the result.

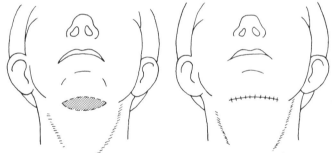

Submental lipectomy corrects a double chin. Shaded portion represents skin to be excised. Final sutures are concealed under the chin.

Generally the standard face lift will do away with wattles and a sagging neck line, but it cannot do much about the presence of the large fat pad under the chin that we call a double chin. Surgeons are aware of the hazards of removing this fat by working under the facial flaps created by rhytidoplasty because of possible damage to the nearby branches of the facial nerve. A safer method is to excise the fatty or subcutaneous tissue situated under the chin—a procedure called a submental lipectomy. A T-shaped or transverse incision is made under the chin, and superfluous skin and fat are removed. The scar heals as a fine line, which, being under the chin, is hidden from direct view. This operation may be performed separately or in conjunction with the rhytidoplasty, depending on the judgment of the surgeon.

Face Lifts in Men

Since hiding scars in the hair-bearing regions of the scalp is given primary consideration in face lifts, the operation in men presents some unique problems. It would be impossible to do a face lift on a man who was completely bald unless he were willing to wear a wig. Even in men with hair, the scars back of the ear must be judiciously placed since most men do not wear their hair long enough to be combed over the ears. However, most men contemplating face lifts are advised to wear their hair longer. The incision in front of the ears is much less of a problem because the majority of men have rather deep creases in that area which serve to conceal the scars.

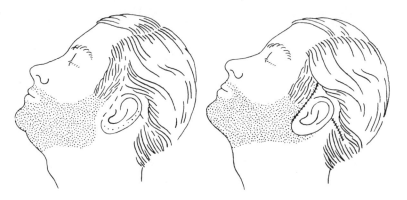

Incision for male face lift is made in hair-bearing skin. Skin is rotated upward and backward and incisions closed.

As in women, the incisions may be started in the hair-bearing scalp in the region of the temples. Some surgeons advocate starting with a horizontal incision from the outside corner of the eye to the ear. But other surgeons frown on this because they feel it may result in an irregular hairline, since the sideburns must be moved back in the face lift. This will narrow or obliterate the strip of hairless skin that is usually present between the inside margin of the sideburn and the ear. When the skin is drawn backward and upward in the tightening process, some of the hair-bearing skin of the cheek will end up behind the lobe of the ear. This hair-bearing skin will continue to grow hair even when it is in its new position and consequently it must be shaved daily. However, it is generally a small area just in back of the earlobe and is not disfiguring. The hair may be removed by electrolysis, if desired. Men planning face lifts must be told about this before surgery. How does Arthur P. feel about this additional shaving chore?

No problem. I'm used to it and it's really just an extra swipe or two with the razor. I was told about it in advance, so it didn't come as a surprise. As of now, I doubt if I'd go to the time and trouble of electrolysis—the hair is not that conspicuous or that much trouble to deal with.

As in all types of surgery, complications can occur. The human body is a wonderfully fashioned and unbelievably complicated organism with incredible ability to repair itself, but it is not like a computer whose reactions can be programmed. Sometimes, in spite of the most ideal conditions—skillful surgery and top-flight hospital care—things can go wrong.

They are rare, but there are always the possibilities of infections, scarring, hair loss, facial-nerve injury, skin sloughs (loss of skin tissue), and hematomas (swellings filled with blood). Another complication could be a result inconsistent with what the patient had in mind. There is an effective treatment for almost all complications.

Hematomas are the most troublesome and frequent complication. Small hematomas are quite common and are spontaneously absorbed within a few weeks. Massive hematomas respond satisfactorily when they are treated promptly. Sometimes they require surgery. Hematomas generally occur within the first 48 hours after surgery.

Infection is extremely rare after a face lift, undoubtedly because of the excellent blood supply in the region. Extensive infections can be treated with appropriate antibiotics.

Heavy scars can occur in face lifts but these too are rare. The weltlike overgrowth called a keloid is difficult to treat but the hypertrophic scar is often improved with time and patience. Superficial x-ray therapy is often useful.

Hair loss occasionally occurs around an incision, particularly in the region of the temples or behind the ear. It is not usually extensive and it is more often temporary than permanent, although it may take up to six months to grow back.

The incisions for a face lift are close to the branches of the nerve that controls the muscles of facial expression. There is risk of injury to one or more branches of this nerve. It rarely happens, but it is possible to injure a nerve, causing paralysis to a part of the face. The greatest risk is to the nerve of the lower lip, the eyelid, or the forehead. Most paralyses clear spontaneously in a few weeks or a few months.

Skin slough, a localized area of dead tissue, is a greatly feared complication. It may be caused by one of a number of conditions that interferes with the blood supply to the operated part. The end result may be an unsightly scar that requires surgical correction. Fortunately, skin sloughs are exceedingly rare.

Complications

After Surgery

When patients regain consciousness after surgery, they will probably find themselves in their hospital beds, and reasonably comfortable. Their heads are encased in a large cocoon-like bandage, with or without drains. The purpose of the bandage is to support the tissues in place, to prevent bleeding under the tissues, and to hold down postoperative swelling. The ears under the bandage are well padded. The patient's face will be swollen and it may or may not be discolored. The large dressing will be kept in place anywhere from 24 to 48 hours before being removed. Many doctors prefer that their patients lie quietly in bed until the dressing is removed, with their heads raised at about a 30-degree angle to keep the swelling to a minimum. After that, small inconspicuous dressings may remain, most of which can be concealed by the patient's hair, or by a wig. Outside of a feeling of numbness and tightness in the face and on the side of the neck below the ears, patients rarely experience any pain. The numbness and tightness may persist for a time, but they will gradually diminish and disappear.

The usual hospital stay for a face lift operation is three or four days. Some patients ask to be discharged the day of or the morning after surgery. This may be allowed if the surgeon feels that the patient's condition permits.

The surgeon determines when the stitches are ready to be removed. Those in front of the ear are the first to be removed because healing in front of the ear, where there is little tension, is always faster than in the back of the ear and the temple regions, where greater tension exists. Generally by the tenth day most or all of the stitches are removed.

There is no hard and fast rule about when people may return to their normal activities. It would depend upon how they look and feel. Some patients have more swelling and discoloration than others, but these symptoms usually subside substantially within five days or so, and by two weeks after the operation most people are presentable. When both face and eyelid surgery are done, the patients should plan on a convalescent period of 14 to 21 days. Patients who live alone should make plans for food and supplies or help from their friends to take care of their needs in case they are housebound for a period of time.

No two people's responses to illness or injury are ever exactly alike. Some patients seem to sail through the aftermath of the face lift with the ease of a sea gull gliding through the air. The passage of time often dilutes and diminishes an unpleasant memory, but Leonard T.'s face lift had been done just five weeks earlier and his account made the operation sound about as traumatic as a pedicure. Leonard is 57 and is with an advertising firm peopled mostly by men and women in their thirties.

I didn't look conspicuously out of place among them, but I didn't mind closing the gap a little. I went into the hospital on a Sunday. Monday was the operation and that day is lost forever. I don't remember a thing. Tuesday I had two of the blackest eyes ever seen outside of a knock-down drag-out street brawl. On Wednesday the big bandage was removed. Some of the stitches were released and others loosened and I went home with no dressings or bandages. I wore dark glasses and was not very swollen, so I don't think I looked too bad. By Saturday all the discoloration in and around my eyes was gone and on Sunday I went to the beach but I did let someone else drive the car, which normally I would not have done. I wore a hat and dark glasses and stayed out of the sun and no one noticed anything unusual. I could have gone back to work that Monday but I indulged myself with an extra week at home.

Leonard's experience is not the usual one and many patients are not quite prepared for the battered, bruised face they take home after a face lift operation. They came into the hospital looking inconspicuously normal and many leave, swollen and distorted, at their very worst. Adele recalls:

I looked an absolute horror, with a swollen face, slitty red swollen eyes, and the black crust around my mouth from the chemical peel. The friend who came to the hospital to take me home walked right by me without recognizing me. I had to tell her who I was.

It is not uncommon for people to go through a period of depression a few days after surgery, similar to the "postpartum blues" experienced by many mothers after childbirth. But in this case, they wonder what madness drove them to have the operation. Some may not be visions of beauty at the moment, but even those people who are not too disfigured may experience the same plummeting spirits. They should try to remember, as they hit their all-time low, that this is not a unique reaction. The best course of action is to take a deep breath, perhaps a tranquilizer, and above all, to have faith that the panic will pass. It always does, sometimes in only a few hours. As Adele says:

I wish I had been better prepared for when the blues hit me. If I had known that this sort of thing happened, I think I would have been able to deal with it a little better. But as it was, I was frantic and inconsolable the whole day ... I must have wept buckets. By evening I was better but it was a dreadful day. I think that every patient should be told this can happen.

And as long as I'm giving advice, the other tidbit I'd like to pass along to people planning this kind of surgery is to avoid as much as possible looking into the mirror for the first few weeks. I did it and it's a big mistake. It only causes needless worry. Stitches don't heal uniformly. The two sides of the face are not completely symmetrical and plastic surgery can't make them so if they're not. All healing is not alike so you mustn't look hypercritically and expect uniform healing. You have to be patient and have confidence in your doctor and the fact that nature will take care of its all coming together.

Recovery Period

Patients are advised not to do any heavy lifting, stretching, bending or straining for a few weeks after a face lift to give the sutures adequate time to heal completely. It could also be advantageous for people to make a conscious effort to cultivate a tranquil expression if they have been in the habit of punctuating their speech with excessive facial contortions. There is also the prohibition against overexposure to the sun. Particularly after facial surgery, excessive sun may interfere with healing. No one should go into the sun for extended periods without the ample protection of good sun-screen creams or lotions on their skins and, for good measure, a broad-brimmed hat on their heads.

Facial makeup can be applied about a week after surgery. There are many tinted cover-up preparations for both men and women that will conceal any slight discolorations that are still present. Patients may comb their hair gently on the fourth day after facial surgery using warm water and a large-toothed comb. Hair may be shampooed on the sixth day. Rollers may be used in the hair if they are put in loosely. Since feeling in the ears may not be quite restored, the drier should be at moderate heat. The hot setting might burn the ears without the patient's being aware. Tinting and coloring of the hair may be done three weeks after surgery. Men may shave their faces lightly, without pulling, seven to ten days following face lifts. Patients may find it advantageous to massage the final scars lightly with moisturizing creams or simple, bland ointments to promote softening and complete healing.

Follow-Up

Following the surgery, doctors see patients in their offices at regular intervals, perhaps once a week for the first month, and then less often. Most of the remaining stitches are generally removed at the first office visit after the surgery. After a period of months—and the length of time is discretionary with the surgeon—the patient is asked to return to the photographer for the "after" photographs. When there are no complications and both doctor and patient are satisfied with the results, the patients are discharged. There is no charge for follow-up visits.

In some cases, however, after a few months have passed and the results are stabilized, the surgeon may wish to make some adjustments. In cosmetic facial surgery, the prudent surgeon

44

prefers to err on the side of underachievement, which can be rectified, rather than to run the risk of causing distortion by doing too much. Where there is a condition that requires attention, the secondary procedure will be performed without charge. The doctor is as eager for a fine result as the patient.

But sometimes a patient's dissatisfaction is based on an unrealistic expectation, in spite of the doctor's having clearly stated at the first consultation what could and could not be achieved. Either the patient forgot what the doctor said or failed to hear it in the first place. This situation has come up even in cases with results that from a technical point of view were superb.

If the doctor feels that nothing more can be done and the patient is still displeased, the patient should seek another opinion from a properly qualified plastic surgeon. In the majority of cases, however, doctor and patient can reach an understanding between them. Adele's situation is relevant:

"I'm thrilled with what was done," she said, "but maybe not a hundred percent happy. I'm thrilled because all that extra stuff around my eyes is gone and for the first time in years I can wear eye makeup. My upper lip is smooth and my lipstick doesn't end up in little grooves on my face as it used to do. My neck is firm and my jowls are gone. I've always had loads of energy but before the operation, even when I wasn't tired, I'd look awful. Now I can feel awful and not look tired.

"But about that hundred percent not happy ..." She pointed to a faint horizontal line that marred ever so slightly the smoothness of her cheeks. "When I asked the doctor about it, he pointed it out on the 'before' photograph. It wasn't so conspicuous before because there were so many other bags and lines. He explained why he couldn't pull up that part of the cheek and I understand." Adele's surgeon has an agreement with his patients that includes any corrective work that needs to be done within a year after the surgery. "He suggested silicone injections for the lines but I'll have to think about that," said Adele. "I have five more months to decide . But let me say this," she added. "In case you're wondering if I'd go through this again, the answer is yes. In ten years, I'll have another face lift if I need it."

Fees

Surgical fees for a face lift range from $1,500 to $5,000. The average fee is about $2,500. A mini-lift ranges from $500 to $1,500, depending on how extensive it is.

The total cost of the face lift operation includes the surgeon's consultation and surgical fees, hospitalization and operating room, the "before and after" photographs, and, if general anesthesia is given, the anesthetist's fee.

45

One Patient's
Experience

Every plastic surgeon knows the frustration of treating patients who, in spite of a technically splendid result, did not achieve the impossible dream they thought the surgery would bring about. Naturally, they blame the doctor. On the other hand, all surgeons have in their files heart-warming and ego-bolstering histories of patients whose ultimate results far exceeded the doctor's expectations. Such a case is Margaret P. and it lends support to the view that cosmetic surgery can indeed be psychiatric therapy performed with a scalpel.

Margaret's silver-blond hair frames a smooth, unlined face and creamy skin. The firm chin line, unwrinkled neck, and bright blue eyes bordered by uncreased lids could belong to a well-preserved and pampered woman in her fifties. Margaret is neither. She is 70 years old and until two years ago worked full time as a psychologist with a social agency while carrying on a small private practice.

Life was pleasant for Margaret. An unsuccessful marriage was long over and forgotten. She shared her apartment with her mother, an extraordinary elderly lady of great intelligence and vitality. The two women were profoundly good friends, mutually admiring each other. Margaret had her work, pleasant associations with friends and colleagues, and the love and support of her mother.

When Margaret was 64, her mother, then 90, died. Margaret's world collapsed. She felt completely alone and abandoned. For an entire year after her mother's death she was plunged into a morass of grief. She functioned on her job, which became the outside perimeter of her life. Severely depressed, she gave up her private practice and refused to see her friends.

Being psychiatrically oriented—she had gone through a period of analysis in addition to her professional training as a psychologist—she realized that she could not go on along this destructive path. Her grief had taken its toll on her face and she felt that her ravaged appearance was not helping her. She sensed that if she looked better, she would feel better about herself. But this created the usual conflict because she had been brought up to believe that one's looks should not be given top priority in life and overconcern with appearance was vain and frivolous.

Support came from an unexpected source when a valued long-time doctor-friend not only encouraged her to take steps to improve her appearance, but went further and recommended her to a plastic surgeon. Margaret is in moderate financial circumstances, but the doctor agreed with her on the wisdom of the expenditure.

Fortunately for Margaret, the surgeon was not only a brilliant technician, but also highly sensitive to the needs of his patient. His support and understanding were to become a pivotal force in Margaret's rehabilitation. Margaret was agreeable to his recommendations for a face lift, eyelid surgery, elevation of the eyebrows, and reshaping and reduction of the lower lip.

The surgery went well. At the end of a month, the swelling and black and blue marks had disappeared except for some slight discoloration around the eyes which was concealed by dark glasses, and Margaret returned to work.

Margaret is a very private person and had never discussed her plans for the operation with any of her colleagues. The time was the end of the summer when vacations are not unusual, and if any of her office associates suspected that her fresh rested look came from other than a splendid vacation, they had the good judgment not to mention it.

But it made no difference to Margaret whether anyone noticed or not. Everything had changed. Her depression vanished and she found herself imbued with a sense of renewal, a resurgence of confidence, and a feeling of her own value as a woman. It seemed to spill over into her work as well, for her office contract was renewed annually for three years past the usual retirement age of 65. "I doubt if that would have happened with my old tired face and the way it made me feel," she said.

Five years after the first operation Margaret returned to the hospital for surgery on her sagging jaw line and neck. The previous surgery had concentrated on the upper part of the face which was as firm as ever but now the chin line and throat needed additional tidying up. Although Margaret is slim, a double chin had developed.

The surgeon performed a submental lipectomy to remove the double chin, and also tightened the skin around the lower part of her face. It was a simple operation and Margaret left the hospital three days later with no telltale discoloration. "I could have gone to a party that same evening," she said. Less than two months after the operation, the small horizontal scar under the chin which provided the escape hatch for the fat pad situated there was scarcely to be seen.

"I know I had the surgery for the right reasons," said Margaret. "It was not a search for youth. I just wanted to feel good about myself ... and I do. Nothing has really changed, but I don't feel inhibited by my age. I've decided to retire from practice and use these bonus years the best way I know how. I don't need the distraction of work any longer. I have a sense of serenity and contentment that comes from within myself that I know I could not have attained with my time-worn face."

FACE LIFT
Before

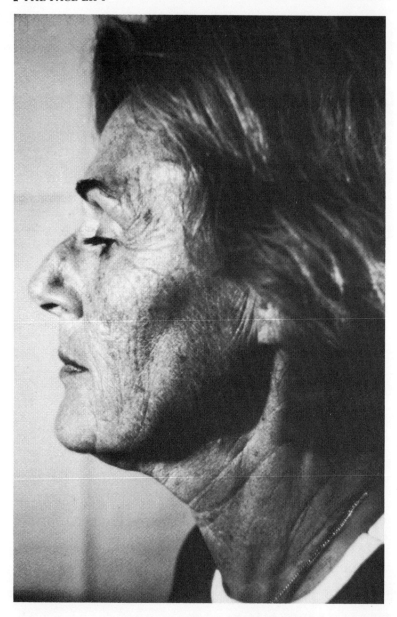

After

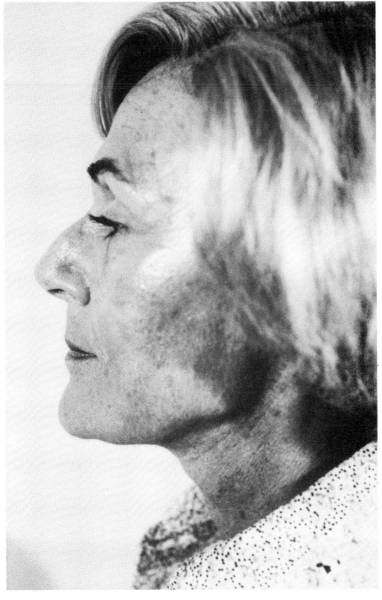

PHOTOGRAPHS COURTESY OF RUDI A. UNTERTHINER, M.D.

49

FACE LIFT
Before

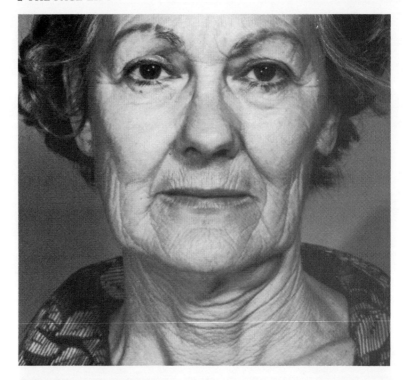

After

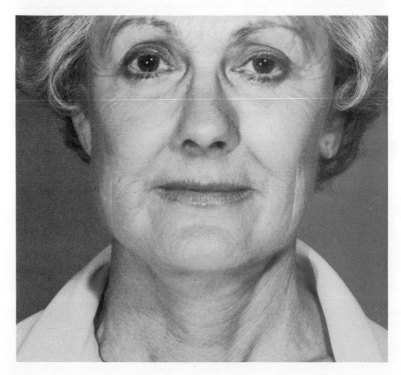

Before

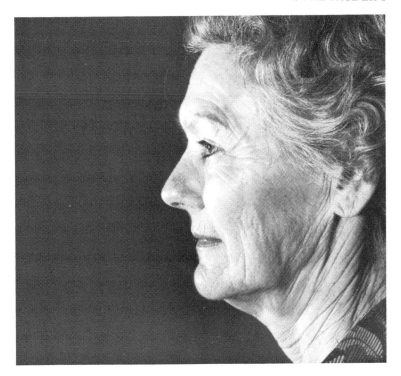

After

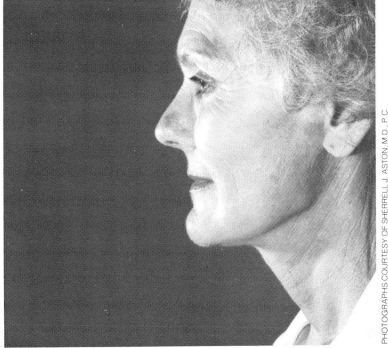

PHOTOGRAPHS COURTESY OF SHERRELL J. ASTON, M.D., P.C.

3
Eyelid Correction

It was not so many years ago that people whose eyes had crepey, sagging eyelids above and bulges and pouches below considered this unattractive condition to be part of the normal course of events. They thought that since it was either a family characteristic or caused by aging, it had to be accepted and endured. Today, however, the correction of this condition by an operation called blepharoplasty has become an everyday occurrence and a surgical procedure approved by the medical profession. It is the most frequently performed of all aesthetic facial operations and can be done by a well-trained plastic surgeon or an eye surgeon with training in aesthetic eye surgery.

The eyes are the single most expressive feature in the human face. They are the first feature that people will observe in each other when they meet. In an otherwise impassive face, the eyes can convey love and warmth. They can smile, twinkle, flash with anger, or by their blank look indicate a mental vacuum. It is interesting that this should be so, for outside of the pupil, whose range of expression is limited to dilating or contracting according to the amount of light to which it is exposed, the eyeball is an unchanging globe. What, then, gives the eyes the ability to convey so much emotion and feeling? It is the tissues surrounding the eyes, the shape of the skin, the lashes and the eyebrows that give them the power to express volumes of feeling.

A plain face can be illuminated by lovely eyes; by the same token, an otherwise youthful face can take on a tired, worn, or even dissipated look when the eyes are surrounded by baggy skin and pouches. It is not difficult, then, to account for the popularity of blepharoplasty or for the fact that it is as frequently performed on men as on women. Unlike a face lift, there has never been a stigma attached to eyelid repair because it often serves a functional purpose in addition to a cosmetic one. Drooping eyelids or excess folds of skin that hood the eyes are not only unsightly but in extreme cases can obscure vision.

Most plastic surgeons agree that there is no single procedure in cosmetic surgery that can have as dramatic an effect in restoring a youthful look to an aging face as blepharoplasty. It is among the most satisfactory of all facial plastic procedures: the recovery time is the shortest and the results the most long-lasting. Once the bags under the eyes are removed, they rarely recur. Since the upper part of the face stretches and sags less than the lower part, eyelid and brow corrections endure longer than face lifts—generally 10 to 15 years. For the rest of the patient's life, the skin around the eyes will be tighter and smoother than it would have been without the surgery. But again, the biological clock does not stop ticking, and the major improvement will lessen as time goes on.

People who must choose between an equally needed blepharoplasty and a face lift because of limited time or money may be advised to have a blepharoplasty, since it will produce the most conspicuous and gratifying results.

A blepharoplasty is also among the most exacting operations in cosmetic surgery, leaving no margin for error. The results are so exposed and open to public gaze that nothing short of complete success can be considered successful.

Early Eyelid Surgery

The first report on surgery of the eyelid goes back almost 1,000 years. It is credited to a man named Avicenna (980-1037) who was court physician and prime minister to different caliphs in Arabia in the late 10th and early 11th centuries. Called "The Prince of Physicians," Avicenna noted that overhanging folds in the upper eyelids impaired vision, and it is believed that he devised ways of removing the excess skin.

Although eyelid surgery was performed over the succeeding centuries, not much was added to the medical literature about it until the late 1700s. In 1818, Carl Ferdinand von Graefe (1787-1840), a professor of surgery at the University of Berlin and founder of modern plastic surgery, introduced the name blepharoplasty to describe the operation. However, his interest in it had nothing to do with its value in enhancing appearance. His concern was with a reconstructive procedure to improve deformities connected with malignancies of the eyelids.

By the mid 1800s, the presence of orbital fat was recognized and described. This is the fat in the bony socket that contains the eyeball—nature's way of providing shock absorbers for the delicate organ. Interest and experimentation in eyelid surgery continued among European surgeons, but the surgery was limited to removal of excess skin of the upper eyelids. Protruding fat was removed from the eyelids only when it was markedly obvious. Aesthetic surgery for baggy eyelids did not really begin until later, but the work of the 19th-Century doctors set the scene for the coming era of eyelid surgery.

Early in the 1900s, a popular operation among European doctors to correct crow's-foot wrinkles at the outside corners of the eyes consisted of excising a small amount of skin at the temple regions and in front of the ears. This is similar to what is known today as a mini-lift. It was strongly criticized by many doctors at that time just as it is now.

By the 1940s, the presence of the fat compartments in the upper and lower eyelids and the necessity of removing them were universally accepted. There have been many variations in the evolution of blepharoplasty from that time until today. A long list of distinguished surgeons have made important contributions to refining the techniques of the operation that have brought it to its present high level.

The eyelids, those movable shades of unbelievable complexity, perform a number of vital functions. They protect the eyes from external injuries and keep bits of foreign matter from entering the eyes; protect the eyes from sudden, blinding light; protect the eyeballs during sleep; and serve to distribute tears over the surface of the eyeball. The tears are essential to the health of the eye: they keep the eyeball moist, dilute any irritants that get into the eye, and wash away foreign particles that have entered the eye. The skin of the upper eyelid is the thinnest in the entire body, permitting the rapid and involuntary opening and closing of the eye. The thinness of the skin and the lack of a layer of fat under it make it a prime prospect for early wrinkling.

The Eyelids

There are two pockets of fatty tissue in the upper lid, but it often appears that there are three because the one nearer the outside corner of the eye—the lateral fat pocket—sometimes seems to be separated into two parts. The fat pocket nearest the nose—the medial fat pocket—gives an inner fullness to the lid at this point.

In the lower lid there are three fat pockets that lie next to one another in the inner, central, and outer thirds of the lid. As a result of the weakening of the membranes that contain them, these fat pockets, known as herniated orbital fat, sometimes protrude forward against the muscle and the skin, causing a generalized bulging—those all-too-familiar pouches—of the lower lid.

Although the fat in the eyelids is called herniated orbital fat, this term is somewhat of a misnomer. It is not like a hernia that occurs in other parts of the body where the hernia actually goes through an opening into the tissues. A true hernia is treated by reinforcing the opening through which it has occurred. But there is rarely any true herniation of the fat in the eyelids into subcutaneous tissues. The "herniated" orbital fat will not respond to tightening a muscle: it cannot be corrected by any means other than removal. The fat pads around the eyes have nothing to do with body weight; they do not vary with either loss or gain and once they are removed they do not recur.

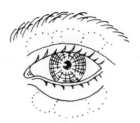

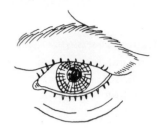

Dotted areas represent pockets of fat under the skin in upper and lower eyelids.

The candidate for eyelid correction has drooping upper lid, pouches under the eye, and drooping eyebrow.

What Causes Baggy Eyelids

Baggy eyelids can occur at any age and from a wide variety of causes. They may reflect the presence of a physical disorder such as an allergy, kidney disease, hypothyroidism, trichinosis, and certain cardiac conditions. But the most common story they tell is one of aging or heredity.

In adolescents or young people, baggy eyelids are usually the result of an overabundance of orbital fat, generally an inherited characteristic, which will appear in many members of the same family. The fat bulges under the eyes may begin to show when the young people are still in their teens and early twenties. The bulges are progressive and should be removed early in their development because with the passage of time they tend to stretch the skin and become increasingly prominent. They are generally more evident below the eye. The upper eyelids may or may not be involved. There is rarely a need to excise skin under the eyes in young people; they need only the removal of fat. This is generally done through some very short incisions and few sutures are required.

After the age of 50, sagging eyelids and pouches around the eyes are a common condition, brought about by the relentless process of aging. The skin has become thinner and lost some of its elasticity. With the diminishing subcutaneous fat and muscle tone, the lines around the eyes become permanent creases. In the upper lid, the excess skin may form an apron that hoods the eyes and there may be ptosis (drooping) of the eyebrow due to muscle weakness. The fat pads may produce a generalized bulging of the lower lid, and the sagging skin may form bags and pouches, or both conditions may be found, one unhappily accentuating the other.

The surgeon must determine whether the condition of the

56

eyelids is caused by a physical disorder, for if so, it would return after the blepharoplasty and the operation would have been useless. There have been any number of cases where people suffering from hypothyroidism were spared an eyelid operation when the proper dosage of thyroid extract made their bags and puffs disappear.

When there is a question about the prospective patient's general health or the possibility of a condition of the eye itself being a complicating factor, the surgeon may request an opinion from the patient's internist or ophthalmologist. It might be noted that chronic glaucoma does not necessarily contraindicate a blepharoplasty.

Stress, anxiety, and tension may also play a part in the formation of the palpebral bags (palpebral is the medical term that means "pertaining to the eyelid"), just as dissipation, overindulgence in alcoholic beverages, and too little sleep can rob the eyes of their smooth-lidded serenity.

On the other hand, there are many baggy-eyed people whose appearance belies their conventional, regulated life style. They are wrongly accused of all manner of excesses and fast living. Michael H., age 52, a textile designer, talks about it:

I'd go to work most mornings looking as if I'd been on an all-night binge, when, in fact, I'd spent a quiet evening at home and gone to bed early. It's one thing to pay the price for carousing, but to take the consequences for an uncommitted sin is something else. But what finally drove me to have eyelid surgery was when the president of my company took me aside and—like a Dutch uncle—suggested that I ought to stop burning the candle at both ends. That did it! I can't tell you what a relief it is to be rid of that tired, dissipated look.

Martha P. went to an eye surgeon, seeking relief from a different kind of accusation. Martha is 52, a doctor's wife, and mother of a college-age son. By her own description, she is a bit dowdy, more than a bit overweight, and a completely happy woman.

I would imagine I was as unlikely looking a patient as ever went looking for cosmetic surgery. I never thought I had an ounce of vanity about my appearance, but you never know, do you? It began when Stephen, my son, came home from college for his first Christmas vacation. I noticed he seemed a little startled when he saw me. He kept asking me how I felt ... and with a note of real concern in his voice. It made me uneasy. And then at dinner when I went into the kitchen to get dessert, I overheard him say to his father, "But how could she be all right and look like that?" At that point I realized what he was talking about. I'd always had deep circles and bags under my eyes—my father's family all had them and I never gave it any thought. I'm in perfect health and I've always had more energy than anyone I know ... and, well, I looked the way I looked. My husband never seemed to mind. But I must confess that Stephen's reaction did shake me up. I took a good look in the mirror and that gave me a glimmer of how I must appear to others. I decided my eyes had to be done. My husband didn't have any objections and he arranged for me to see a surgeon. The next month I had a blepharoplasty—upper and lower lids. Without telling Stephen, of course. When he came home for spring vacation, there I was, looking better than I had for years, eyes all ironed out and my face in one piece again. Did Stephen notice anything different? Certainly not. But he didn't ask me how I was feeling, either.

The Blepharoplasty	The ultimate aim of a blepharoplasty is to remove the excess skin in the upper eyelids, to smooth out the eyelids, to remove the bags under the eyes, and, most important, to achieve a natural expression around the eyes. Since no two faces are exactly alike, each operation must be tailored individually to the patient's requirements and no single surgical technique will do for everyone. The surgeon must be creative and resourceful in planning precisely what has to be done to achieve the desired result.

In some cases, where fallen eyebrows have exaggerated the excess skin in the upper eyelid, the removal of the eyelid skin alone will not result in full improvement. The eyebrows may also require lifting. The surgeon must decide on the amount of dropping of the eyebrow; the amount of excess skin and protruding fat on the upper eyelid that must be removed; the amount and type of excess skin and the amount and distribution of fat on the lower eyelid that must be dealt with.

In addition to improving the appearance of the eyes, a blepharoplasty is also performed for the functional purpose of correcting ptosis—a drooping of the upper eyelid. This condition may be caused by a weakness of the muscle that raises and lowers the eyelid, or by an injury. Some patients with pronounced ptosis are obliged to tilt their heads backward to get a full field of vision.

Occasionally found on the upper and lower eyelids near the inside corners of the eyes are small, velvety, yellowish deposits of xanthomas. They are benign in character and sometimes associated with one of a number of physical disorders, high blood cholesterol among them. Small, discrete xanthomas are easily removed (Chapter 7).

When very large skin bags are present, it may be necessary to do the operation in two procedures, spaced several months apart, in order to determine accurately the exact amount of skin to be excised.

To avoid disappointment, the patient should be made aware of what blepharoplasty cannot accomplish. It cannot eliminate bulges, hollows, or bags of skin in the cheek area below the eyelid itself. It will improve many of the wrinkles and folds around the eyes when the face is in repose, but it cannot eradicate the horizontal lines that appear around the eyes when the face is animated, as in frowning or laughing. Excessively wrinkled skin around the eyelids will be improved, but it cannot be smoothed out completely as you would iron a rumpled sheet. In some cases, fine wrinkles show up after a blepharoplasty because removing bulging fat releases the tension that tends to stretch the eyelid skin. These fine wrinkles can sometimes be treated with a chemical peel (Chapter 7).

What Blepharoplasty Cannot Do

As in all cosmetic surgery, photographs must be taken in advance of the operation. They are particularly important in the eyelid operation because sometimes certain problems, such as a marked discrepancy between the sizes of the bulges under the eyes that may not have been obvious during the physical examination of the patient, become apparent in a photograph.

Preoperative Procedures

If the operation is being done in a hospital, it is customary for the patient to be admitted the day before the surgery. There has been a recent trend for more of these operations to be done in the doctor's office or in an outpatient surgical facility. This has come about because of the ever-rising hospital costs and the refusal of Blue Cross (in some states) to reimburse for cosmetic surgery. The night before surgery, the patients wash their faces thoroughly with an antibacterial soap such as pHisoHex.

Patients are generally advised not to take aspirin or any medication containing salicylates for two weeks before and after surgery, since aspirin can promote bleeding. Tylenol or Datril are recommended as substitutes. Women are advised to discontinue any hormone medication for ten days to two weeks prior to surgery.

Blepharoplasty can be done under general or local anesthesia. The choice varies with each surgeon, with local anesthesia the choice for most. Local anesthesia is usually administered with epinephrine (adrenalin). This helps to separate the tissue layers and also to stop bleeding. Local anesthesia is sometimes supplemented with intravenous Valium given during the course of the operation. Pain is negligible and patients have little recollection of the operation.

Anesthesia

The order in which the lids are done is a matter of choice with the surgeon. Some prefer to operate on the lower lids first be-

Surgical Procedure

cause they demand the greatest amount of attention, time, and skill. The operation for both upper and lower lids takes between 1½ and 2 hours. The upper eyelids alone take about half an hour.

Upper Eyelids

Before the patient is anesthetized, the surgeon outlines the amount of skin to be removed from the upper eyelid, using a brightly colored marking pen. In order to determine the amount of tissue that needs to be trimmed, the patient is asked to open and close the eyes a few times. If the excess skin is located primarily in the central portion of the upper lid, only an elliptical area of skin may need to be removed. But if there is a great deal of loose tissue around the outer corners of the eyes, as is more often the case, a longer incision that ends in the natural crow's-foot wrinkles will be made. The incision marks are carefully placed so that the resulting scar will fall within the normal skin creases when the eyes are open. The lowermost incision line becomes the final suture line.

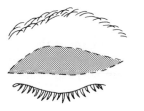

Left: For upper eyelid correction, a wedge of skin is removed (shaded area).

Right: After the skin is removed, the wound is sutured.

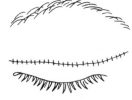

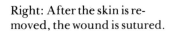

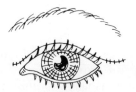

Left: The scar is concealed in the natural crease of the eyelid.

After the anesthetic is administered, the predetermined amount of excess skin is removed. Once this skin is excised, the accumulation of fat lying beneath the muscle is easily identified and removed. In young people, there is generally no excess skin to be excised, but in the middle-aged and older, both skin and fat must be taken care of. Throughout the operation, the surgeon carefully tracks down and seals off all bleeding points. If ptosis of the eyelid is present, it is corrected at this time by a separate procedure that involves the muscles that control the eyelid. Muscle fibers are reunited and the incision is closed with fine sutures.

Lower Eyelids

The lower eyelid is the most challenging part of cosmetic blepharoplasty. Unlike the upper lid where the skin tends to stretch with time, the removal of too much skin of the lower lid can cause it to turn out at the edge, producing a disfiguring condition called an ectropion, or it may cause excessive exposure of the whites of the eye (sclera) below the pupil. Surgeons are deliberately conservative when working on the lower lid for it is easier to correct a condition if too little skin has been taken than to restore it if too much was removed.

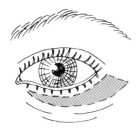
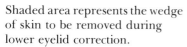
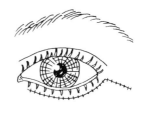

Shaded area represents the wedge of skin to be removed during lower eyelid correction.

Final sutures are concealed by lower eyelashes and natural creases at corner of the eye.

The surgeon marks off the skin to be removed from the lower lid. The incision parallels the lower lid margin from the inner corner of the eye to slightly past the outer corner, curving into one of the crow's-foot lines at the outside corner of the eye. The final thin scar will be almost invisible and further concealed by the lower eyelashes. After the skin has been incised, the lower lid will be undermined. The fibers in the muscle surrounding the eyelids are gently separated so that the fat pockets can be seen. The surgeon must use the most critical judgment in removing the fat because if too much is taken a hollow will be created below the lid, and there is little cosmetic advantage in exchanging a hollow for a bulge. Throughout the surgery, every bleeding point is sealed to avoid hematoma (a collection of blood within the tissues), which can prolong convalescence. After excising the fat from the three pockets, the surgeon makes the necessary repairs to the underlying tissues and muscle. Then the skin is pulled gently upward, the excess skin trimmed away, and the incision closed with fine sutures.

**Correction of
Dropped
Eyebrows**

Dropping of the brows can occur with the aging process. The purpose of the eyebrow lift is to return the eyebrows to their original position which gives the face a more youthful appearance. They are elevated by excising an ellipse of forehead skin directly above and along the length of the eyebrow. The greater the amount of skin that is excised, the higher the brow will be lifted. The incision is placed so that the final scar will lie as close to the hair of the eyebrow as possible.

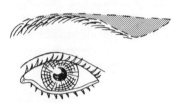

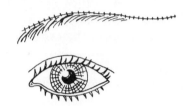

To raise a drooping eyebrow, an ellipse of skin is removed.

Final sutures leave a scar as close to the eyebrow as possible.

However, in spite of the surgeon's best efforts, the scar is not always successfully concealed and patients must be made aware that it may remain visible after healing is complete. In some patients the eyebrow lift is highly successful, but where it is not, it can cause disappointment.

A pressure dressing is applied to the incisions and held in place with a bandage around the head. Stitches are removed in a few days and replaced with small adhesive strips to prevent scar spreading. The brow area may feel numb for a time, but this is transitory and gradually full feeling returns. Eyebrow correction may be done at the same time as the blepharoplasty.

**After
the Operation**

Some surgeons, but not all, do not bandage the eyes after a blepharoplasty because many patients find it frightening and claustrophobic. They feel that while there might be some value in using a moderate-pressure dressing for the first few hours following surgery to control oozing, swelling, and hematoma, patients seem to do very well without it. The decision whether or not to bandage the eyes is best left to the surgeon. In standard postoperative procedure, the eyes are well lubricated with a bland ophthalmic ointment, and sterile ice compresses are applied for the remainder of the day, or longer if the patient finds it comforting. The ice packs will not prevent swelling or discoloration, but they will help to minimize it.

Some patients complain of interference with vision for a few hours or a day after surgery, but this generally passes quickly and most people are comfortable reading or watching television by the second or third day after the operation.

There is usually no severe pain after eyelid surgery, but as might be expected, the eyes feel uncomfortable and tight. This tightness could persist for a period of months, but as the skin of the upper eyelid stretches, it lessens and gradually passes.

Robert L., a slim, highly tense 45-year-old man, quick in movement and in speech, has a comment about eye bandaging after blepharoplasty, but he obviously does not represent a majority opinion:

I don't know why anyone would be upset about having their eyes bandaged after this operation. Nobody in the whole world could have been more nervous about this surgery than I was. It took me five years to get up the courage to have it done, even though I had had huge bags under my eyes ever since I was in my middle thirties. But it wasn't until my left eye began to droop so low it interfered with my vision that I knew I couldn't postpone it any longer. You know how Jerry Lewis drops one eyelid when he wants to be funny? That's how I looked—except I wasn't trying to be funny.

Anyway, my doctor had told me he preferred that my eyes be bandaged after the operation so I was prepared for it when I woke up in my room after the operation was over. In a way it was comforting ... nothing to do except lie quietly and relax. No hardship—I was pretty well sedated the whole day and I slept through most of it. The bandages were removed the following morning and when I took a look at my slitty, swollen, discolored eyes, I suggested that they put the bandages back on.

Recovery Period

For the first few days after surgery, there is usually swelling and discoloration, which in some patients may be mild. The eyes may also water a bit, but generally by the tenth postoperative day, swelling, discoloration, and watering of the eyes have begun to diminish noticeably. The intensity of the aftereffects varies with the individual patient and the extent of the surgery. Some patients feel able to return to normal activities within a few days after surgery, their eyes covered by dark glasses. Dark glasses can be worn immediately after surgery and contact lenses may be inserted within a week to ten days later, provided the eyes are not red or the eyelids swollen.

Stitches are removed beginning with the second day after the operation, at the discretion of the doctor. This may be done either in the hospital before the patient is discharged, or in the doctor's office.

Eye makeup may usually be used about five days after the removal of the last sutures. This includes mascara, eye shadow, and artificial eyelashes. Patients should be careful not to tug at the eyelids, because with early removal of the sutures, pulling could cause the skin edges to separate. Eye makeup should be removed gently with oiled eye-makeup-remover pads. Any remaining spots of discoloration around the eyes may be concealed with covering makeup.

Patients should avoid the direct rays of the sun for a few months following blepharoplasty. The sun's rays can interfere with healing. By two or three months after the operation, the scars in most people will have merged with the natural lines above and below the eyes and will scarcely be seen. The thin skin of the lids generally heals well and with little signs of the incision. The scars that extend beyond the eyebrows and lids may take more time to fade and may not be as fine.

Complications Most of the complications of blepharoplasty are temporary. They are usually self-limiting and generally appear almost immediately after surgery.

As in all facial surgery, there is always danger of hematoma, swellings filled with blood, but fortunately permanent damage or serious problems resulting from hematomas are unusual. Its management depends upon where it occurs and how severe it is.

Infections rarely occur following eye surgery because of the rich blood supply to this region. When it does occur, it can be treated with the appropriate antibiotic.

Epiphora is excessive tearing from the eyes. It is common in the first 48 hours after surgery but it may persist for a longer period. It is usually caused by swelling of the skin, distortion of the tear-drainage system, or distortion of the lid margins. When healing is complete, the epiphora usually disappears.

Diplopia, or double vision, may occur during the first few hours or days following surgery. It may be caused by temporary muscle disturbances, reaction to the wound, or swelling of the conjunctiva, which is the delicate membrane that lines the eyelids and covers the front of the eyeballs.

Lagophthalmos, also called hare's eye (*lagōs* is hare in Greek) is the inability to close the eyes completely and is a common complaint during the period immediately following the operation. It may result from the excision of too much skin from the upper eyelids, but this rarely happens. When the eyelid is unable to close tightly, it cannot perform its function of distributing the tears over the eyeball, and the eyeball becomes dry and irritated. In most cases, the eyelid skin stretches and the condition corrects itself in a matter of weeks or months. Until that occurs, there are specific drops and ointments for day and night use that relieve the irritation.

Ectropion is one of the more disturbing complications following blepharoplasty. It can be caused by too much skin being excised from the lower lid, causing the eyelid to turn out at the

64

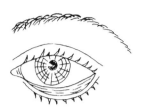

Ectropion is a turning out of the eyelid.

edge. The surgeon gives top priority to avoiding this complication by judicious, conservative excision of the skin of the lower lid. It is quite common for the lower lid to show a light, downward pull after blepharoplasty because of wound reaction. However, this usually subsides within the first few weeks although it is possible in unusual cases for it to persist for several months. This can happen following the removal of very large fat pockets or when the skin is thicker than normal. Temporary ectropion can also be caused by a small hematoma of the wound or excessive swelling of the conjunctiva. It subsides as the hematoma and the swelling subside.

Ectropion that occurs from the removal of too much skin requires reconstruction with skin grafts. Ectropion in older people caused by the relaxation of eyelid tissue requires corrective surgery to the eyelid itself.

Small areas of thickening in the scars can occur, particularly when extensive undermining of the lid has been done. These generally resolve themselves after a period of time. In some cases, injection of a very small amount of steroid compounds in the scar areas will hasten their improvement.

There have been cases of blindness reported following blepharoplasty, but the cases reported did not include information about the condition of the eyes before the surgery, so valid conclusions cannot be drawn. In view of the hundreds of thousands of blepharoplasties performed each year and the rarity of reports of similar incidents, it is possible that these tragedies could have been coincidental to the surgery.

Cathleen P. talks about her experiences following a blepharoplasty, performed ten months earlier:

A Patient's Experience

It was an uneventful operation and I suppose I had an uneventful recovery, although there were a few complications afterward. Everyone says it is a painless operation, and I truly don't remember having any pain ... except that I vaguely recall hearing myself say "Ouch" at one point during the operation—so I imagine I must have felt something, even if I don't remember it.

65

The day after the operation I had double vision so I didn't try to read or watch TV. I was awfully glad I had my transistor radio with me in the hospital. I think it's a good idea for anyone going into the hospital for eyelid surgery to take a radio with them. Music and news are pleasant diversions. The double vision was gone by the next day and I could focus properly when I went home.

And then for a few months after the operation, my eyes didn't close completely and they felt teary and irritated. My doctor gave me some drops—one for day and one for night—and they helped enormously. After a while the eyelids stretched and closed as they were supposed to, so I didn't have any more trouble with that.

But it took almost six months before I felt my eyes really belonged to me. After the operation, they were much larger and rounder than before— half of them had been hidden under the crepey lids, you know—and the new eyes seemed sort of ... well, glary ... and they were tight ... but now they are perfectly comfortable and they're all mine and I couldn't be happier.

Follow-Up Visits
Following the surgery, the patient goes to the doctor's office for removal of stitches and follow-up examination. The patient will be expected to return at intervals, at the discretion of the doctor, until the doctor is assured that all is well and nothing more needs to be done. At that time the surgeon will ask the patient to return to the photographer for the "after" pictures. There is no charge for follow-up visits.

Fees
Surgeon's fees for a blepharoplasty range from $1,000 to $2,000. When only the upper or lower eyelids require surgery, the fee is proportionately less. Some cosmetic surgeons charge $600 to $800 for upper eyelids and the same for lower, depending on how much needs to be done.

Added to the surgeon's fee is the cost of the "before and after" photographs ($35 to $45), hospitalization, and anesthetist ($300 to $600), if the operation is done under general anesthesia. If the operation is done in the surgeon's office, there are no hospitalization or anesthesia costs.

The Oriental Eye
Since World War I, operations to "Westernize" the Oriental eye have become the most popular of all cosmetic surgical procedures in the Far East. This trend has probably been stimulated by increasing interest in and identification with Western clothes, cosmetics, films, books, and music. Remodeling the Oriental eye to the Occidental form is a simple 20-minute operation in the Far East. It is said that in Tokyo alone it is performed on more than a quarter of a million people each year.

The Oriental eye is characterized by the absence of the horizontal skin fold, known as the superior palpebral fold, in the upper eyelid. The lid hangs down like a thick drape, giving the eye a hooded and rather expressionless quality. Some Orientals refer to the eyes without the fold as the "single eye" and the eye with the fold as the "double eye." The "single eye" is a dominant hereditary trait and appears in about 50 percent of Orientals.

There are several anatomical differences between the Oriental and Western eye. There is more skin and fat in the upper lid of the Oriental eye than in the Caucasian. But the most important difference is in the foreshortened levator muscle in the Oriental eye. This is the muscle that elevates the eyelid. In Caucasians and blacks, the muscle is longer and its fiber extensions are attached to the skin of the lid, whereas in the Oriental eye, the muscle fibers do not reach the skin. It is the attachment of the end fibers of the levator muscle to the skin of the eyelid that forms the palpebral fold. Also present in about 50 percent of Orientals is a fold of skin called the epicanthal fold that covers part of the inner corner of the eye. The epicanthus usually begins in the upper lid, follows a crescent-shaped course around the inner corner and ends in the lower lid or along the nose.

There are a number of different techniques employed in transforming the Oriental eye. The simplest procedure, used in outpatient clinics and offices throughout the Orient, is suitable for the younger age group in whom there is a minimum of excess fat and skin. The levator muscle is connected to the eyelid skin by three or four sutures placed on the undersurface of the eyelid. They are left for 10 or 12 days so that adhesions will develop, and then removed. Or the sutures can be inserted in such a way that they are actually pulled beneath the skin and remain permanently. Excess fat in the eyelid is excised through a small puncture in the upper lid. If there is a considerable amount of fat, a larger incision would be required for removal.

The Operation

An advantage of this technique is that it is reversible. Adjustments can be made if the sutures are not placed in exactly the right position and the palpebral folds do not match. In such a situation, the sutures are removed and after an interval of a few weeks, the operation is repeated.

A more radical approach is indicated for the Oriental eye that is noticeably puffy and has more skin and fat. The surgical procedure in this instance would be along the lines of the routine blepharoplasty in the Caucasian eye, with special attention given to attaching the fibers of the levator muscle to the skin. Excess skin and fat in the lower lids would be corrected at the same time as the upper lid repair.

The operation to correct the epicanthal fold is a delicate one.

67

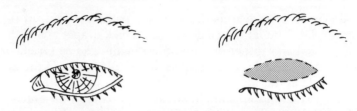

The Oriental eye lacks the horizontal fold. To correct it, an upper lid incision is made and excess fat is removed.

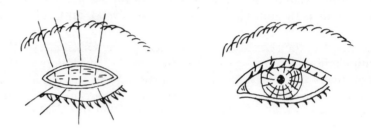

Vertical sutures connect levator muscle with upper and lower edges of eyelid skin. Attaching the levator muscle to the skin creates the desired fold in the upper eyelid.

Removing the skin from the corner of the eye could cause scarring or increase the deformity. Also, Orientals have a tendency to form keloids and the surgeon would have to determine the healing pattern of the skin in advance. Removing the epicanthal fold is best handled by a procedure called a Z-plasty in which the skin at the corner of the eye is redistributed by transferring the upper and lower triangular flaps.

Postoperative Procedure

In the Asian countries, patients leave the doctor's office shortly after the suture construction of a palpebral fold. Generally they see the doctor twice a week for a month or more. Most of the patients are able to return to work the day after surgery.

When this procedure is performed in a hospital in the Western world, the usual hospital two-day stay is observed.

Postoperative results from the more extensive operation are similar to those of a regular blepharoplasty. The operation is usually done in a hospital and requires a two-day stay. Swelling and discoloration may follow as in most eyelid surgery.

Fees

In the United States, the fee range for "Westernizing" the Oriental eye is the same as for the usual upper eyelid blepharoplasty, about $600 to $800. The more extensive procedure would cost the same as for the standard upper and lower eyelid blepharoplasty, ranging from $1,000 to $2,000.

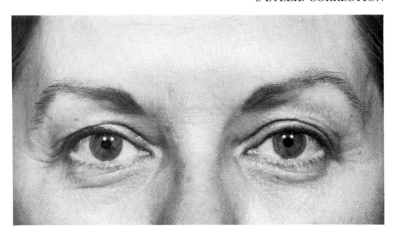

**UPPER AND
LOWER EYELID
CORRECTION**
Before

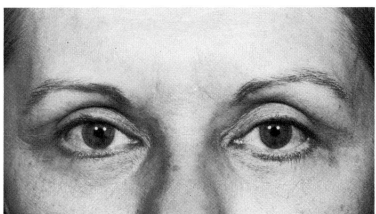

After

PHOTOGRAPHS COURTESY OF SHERRELL J. ASTON, M.D., P.C.

UPPER AND LOWER
EYELID
CORRECTION
Before

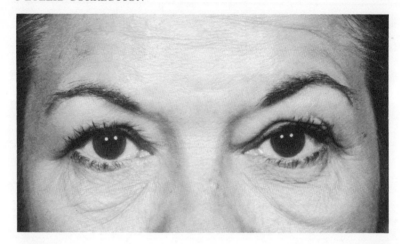

After

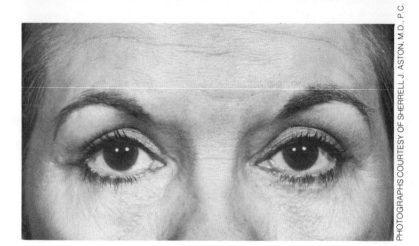

PHOTOGRAPHS COURTESY OF SHERRELL J. ASTON, M.D., P.C.

4
Reconstruction of the Nose

The nose, a hollow pyramid of bone, cartilage, muscle, skin, and mucous membrane, is the most conspicuous feature of the human face; rhinoplasty, the operation to correct it aesthetically and functionally, occupies a similar position of prominence in the hierarchy of cosmetic operations. More than half of all plastic-surgical procedures are performed on the nose and most plastic surgeons agree that it is the most demanding and exacting of all cosmetic facial surgery, drawing upon the surgeon's most highly developed sense of aesthetics as well as great technical skill. The nasal structures must be altered without interfering with their functioning. Rhinoplasty can diminish, straighten, build up, lengthen, shorten, or uptilt a nose. It can help to alleviate a malfunction in breathing, in the sense of smell, and in speaking. And since almost all procedures are performed from inside the nose, there are generally no telltale scars or marks of surgical sutures left behind.

The ultimate aim of a successful rhinoplasty is not a perfect nose but one that is in harmony and balance with the rest of the face and gives no evidence that surgery was ever done. In the words of one of New York City's leading rhinoplastic surgeons, "We try not to make a nose; we try to make a face."

To achieve this, the surgeon must decide on what seems most appropriate for the patient and the best way to go about getting that result. The decision on the height of the bridge of the nose will determine its character; what is done with the nasal tip will add or detract from a successful result. Even the patient's height must be considered in thinking about the shape of the nose; a marked uptilt on tall persons may not be desirable since they already have most people looking up at their nostrils, whereas short or average height people can carry an uptilted nose more gracefully. The correction of a nose that needs just a fraction of improvement requires extreme precision and unerring judgment. There is only the slimmest margin between how much should be removed and how much should be left. Lengthening a nose that was made too short is a more difficult problem than shortening a nose left a bit too long. Rhinoplasty has been described as the "surgery of millimeters," and unlike almost any other cosmetic operation, it is performed within a tightly restricted surgical area.

But all plastic surgeons, no matter how experienced and skillful, face elements beyond their control in each operation they perform. Their technique and aesthetic sense are important, but whatever they do will be limited by the type of nose the patient presents, the thickness of the patient's skin, and the shape and size of the face to which the nose must be fitted. A nose tip that is thick and bulky can never be sculpted into the nose tip with the chiseled look so widely admired. Surgeons can reshape cartilage and bone, but they cannot change the quality of the skin. The final result will also be affected by the healing ability of the patient and the course of the convalescence. Identical twins could each undergo surgery of the nose and each would have a different result.

It cannot be claimed that every patient who has had a rhinoplasty is happy or satisfied; as in all surgery there will be indifferent, even bad results and always there are patients whose expectations could never be realized. But on the other hand there are countless cases of dramatic successes—shy, mousy young girls who blossomed into self-confident beauties when a badly proportioned nose was altered; frustrated women imbued with a sense of renewal and energy because of their pleasing new image; and men of all ages, their self-assurance bolstered by their improved appearance, who found themselves better able to cope with their problems.

Rhinoplasty can be performed by a general plastic surgeon or an otolaryngologist (ear, nose, and throat specialist) who specializes in plastic surgery.

The popularity of rhinoplasty as a cosmetic procedure may be a minor phenomenon of the 20th Century, but plastic surgery of the nose goes back to the early days of recorded history. Historians cite the existence of Egyptian hieroglyphics and ancient Indian writings that indicate that plastic surgery of the nose was performed in India and Egypt between 2500 B.C. and 600 B.C.

An Ancient Art

The reconstruction of the nose using a skin graft was described in a book written in India over 2,000 years ago. At that time, amputation of the nose was a commonly inflicted punishment for adultery and criminal behavior. Whether such a conspicuous punishment achieved its purpose in humiliating the wrongdoer and acting as a warning to others is questionable. The surgery to rehabilitate the victims was carried out by a caste of Hindu potters, the Camaas. The art was closely guarded and passed from father to son for hundreds of years and they did not appear to run short of noses to restore. The operation took about one and a half hours and was performed with a razor.

The nose was refashioned with a skin graft taken from the patient's cheek, or more often, the forehead. The Hindus of that time apparently recognized that the skin of the forehead more nearly matches that of the nose in color and texture than skin from any other part of the body. A segment of skin, the size and shape of the nose, was separated on three sides from its original position and rotated down to cover the nose wound. The fourth side was left attached to the forehead to assure a blood supply and was detached several weeks later after the skin flap had "taken." The wound on the forehead was then grafted with skin from another part of the body. This method of reconstruction became known as the Indian method, although it was used in Egypt and in the Middle East during the same period.

It is interesting to note that the technique of building a missing or partially absent nose that is in use today is basically the same, although the results must be quite different. The Hindus had to rely on formation of scar tissue to give the nose a degree of firmness; today, a fragment of bone, rib cartilage, or silicone is used as a framework for the nose.

Through uncertain channels—perhaps some wandering Indian fakirs—knowledge of the Indian method reached a Sicilian family of plastic surgeons, the Brancas of Catania, in the 15th Century. They practiced nose reconstruction using carefully guarded secret techniques that they passed from one generation to another. People from all over Europe came to them for repairs on noses lost or distorted in wars or in duels or destroyed by leprosy. One of the members of the Branca family, Antonio, devised a new method of using a skin graft from the upper arm instead of the forehead for nasal reconstruction. This became known as the Italian method.

In 1597, Gaspare Tagliacozzi, a young surgeon in Bologna, revived the operation of rhinoplasty, which had been in the hands of the Brancas for the two preceding centuries. He was severely abused and opposed by most surgeons for this. Among them was Ambroise Paré, the barber-surgeon who was the cherished subject of four 16th-Century French kings. The churchmen of that time regarded such operations as meddling with the handiwork of God. Deformities were the will of the Divine Power and were best left alone, they said. Censure followed Tagliacozzi to the grave, for his remains were exhumed from the convent where he was buried and transferred to unconsecrated ground.

Between the 16th and 18th centuries, nasal reconstruction lay dormant in Europe, while in India the relatively unchanged ancient art continued to flourish. But in 1816, Joseph Constantine Carpue, an English surgeon, revived the Indian method of rhinoplasty to restore the nose of an English officer. His success with this case touched off a wellspring of interest in plastic surgery, and from that point on, many of the great surgeons in Europe began to make important contributions to the field of nasal surgery.

The first detailed accounts of nose reduction without external incisions were published in the late 1890s. The techniques of one of the innovators of this procedure, a German surgeon named Dr. Jacques Joseph, has formed the basis for modern rhinoplasty. Dr. Joseph is known as the father of rhinoplastic surgery. His techniques were expanded and developed by the demands of World War II, and in the past two decades there has been a further wave of surgical advances, enriched by the contributions of gifted surgeons from many part of the world.

Plastic surgery had its beginnings in the reconstruction of noses that were damaged by accident, sickness, or congenital deformities. Cosmetic rhinoplasty is a comparatively recent development, starting within the present century.

The Nose

Of prime interest to the plastic surgeon are the nasal skin, the nasal lining, and the nasal skeleton. The skin of the upper portion of the nose is thin, pliable, and easily movable over the underlying bone. The skin of the lower third of the nose is thicker, adheres closely to the underlying cartilage, and is full of sebaceous glands. It does not have the elasticity of the skin of the upper part of the nose. The thickness of this skin varies greatly from person to person, but it is not matched exactly by skin from any other part of the body. Thin-skinned noses generally produce fine aesthetic results in rhinoplasty for the thin skin easily hugs the newly fashioned framework of the nose.

The exterior structure of the nose forms a projecting pyramid from its root (the bridge of the nose) to the base of the columella (the column of flesh that connects the nose to the upper lip). The nose is roofed by paired nasal bones and two pairs of cartilages—the upper lateral and the lower lateral. The lower lateral cartilage forms the nose tip and curves around the nostrils, forming the wings, or alae, of the nose.

The interior of the nose is divided into two chambers by the nasal septum, a partition formed of bone and cartilage. These nasal chambers, or cavities, are lined with mucous membrane. The two openings in the nose, the nostrils, form passageways that carry air to the back of the throat and then to the lungs. The

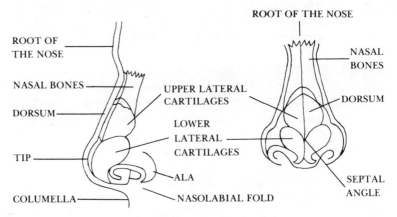

ROOT OF THE NOSE

ROOT OF
THE NOSE

NASAL
BONES

NASAL BONES

UPPER LATERAL
CARTILAGES

DORSUM

DORSUM

LOWER
LATERAL
CARTILAGES

TIP

ALA

SEPTAL
ANGLE

COLUMELLA

NASOLABIAL FOLD

ANATOMY OF THE NOSE

nose performs the important function of warming, moistening, and filtering that air. The nasal cavity can be an extraordinarily effective air conditioner. But in some people, the septum may be deviated or thickened, thus partially or completely blocking one or both nasal passages. This is called a deviated septum and can cause the discomfort of a nasal drip or difficulty in breathing. Not an uncommon condition, it is one that brings many patients to the offices of plastic surgeons and nose and throat specialists. It has been observed that noses that show irregularities on the outside often conceal irregularities on the inside. The deviated septum can be corrected during rhinoplasty.

A deviated septum, besides being aesthetically unpleasing, can interfere with breathing.

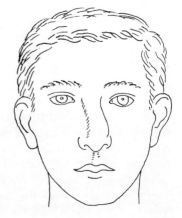

The nose changes more than any other feature from birth onward. The shape of an infant's or small child's eyes and mouth usually casts a shadow of the shape of things to come, but the broad, flat-bridged little protuberance in the middle of the face bears small resemblance to the finished product that will make itself known 14 or 15 years hence. The full-grown nose may be about three times its original length. The unwelcome embellishments such as bumps and humps—those not caused by injury—do not usually appear until the initial growth periods have passed. This could be about 12 or 13 for girls and 14 or 15 for boys.

But even after the middle or late teens when the nose has stopped growing, changes continue to take place in the nose. The relentless process of aging, with the accompanying loss of skin elasticity and muscular framework, aided by the pull of gravity, tends to elongate the nose in the later years. There is also a drooping of the nasal tip. These processes are often arrested in noses that have had rhinoplasty because of the formation of scar tissue that holds the skin and stiffens the structure of the nose.

Age. The minimum age for girls contemplating nose correction operations is at least two full years after the onset of menstruation—no earlier than 15 or 16. Boys mature later than girls, so the recommended age would be delayed to the late teens. The essential consideration in choosing the time for surgery for teenagers is that the nasal bone growth has been completed and the lower lateral cartilages of the nose have attained their maximum degree of firmness. The surgeon is in the best position to judge whether the young person is sufficiently developed for the operation, or whether a delay is advisable.

Physical Considerations

However, there are some situations where young people may require nasal surgery earlier and it would be unwise to wait. For instance, it could be harmful to neglect a nasal obstruction that interfered with breathing. In such a case, limited surgery to the nasal septum would be indicated, but the cosmetic surgery should be postponed until the patient is older.

There is no age limit for rhinoplasty at the other end of the spectrum if the patient is in good physical and mental health. Surgeons report excellent results in well-motivated patients in their late sixties or even older. A doctor tells of such a case:

I was very doubtful of Mrs. A. when she came to see me. She had a valid complaint—she had a large, unattractive nose with a hump and an overhanging tip, but she was obviously in her early seventies, even if she didn't admit to quite all of that . . . . I think she said she was 68. But it seemed to me that she should have made peace with her nose after all those years.

I questioned her about why at this time in her life she wanted an operation on her nose. She said that ever since she was a young woman she had envied a younger sister who had a small, well-shaped nose, and was much prettier than she.

77

I think I should explain that you have to be most cautious about accepting older patients for rhinoplasty. People who have lived with the same nose for a long time often have a great deal of trouble getting accustomed to their new appearance and some never make it. What they see in the mirror is not the same as their self-image and this can be most disturbing emotionally. Young people are more adaptable, maybe because they haven't lived with their faces that long. I've had patients come to see me—and I might have been the third, fourth, or even fifth doctor they'd seen—asking to have the nose restored to its former size and shape.

So Mrs. A.'s competitive feeling about her sister's nose didn't seem to me to be enough of a reason to take her on as a patient. But then she convinced me. She told me that her husband had offered her a fur coat as an anniversary present and she persuaded him that instead of a new coat, what she really wanted was a new nose.

That made up my mind. I decided that any woman who would choose a nose over a fur coat had to have given the matter a lot of careful thought and was sure of what she wanted.

Her first words after the surgery when she saw herself in the mirror were, "Oh Doctor, it's smaller and prettier than my sister's!"

This was a few years ago. I hope she is still around, enjoying her nose. Come to think of it, the fur coat might have gotten shabby by now.

Health. In addition to the usual concern with the patient's general condition and the presence of a chronic disorder that might interfere with healing, there are specific disorders that are particularly pertinent to rhinoplasty. If there is a family history of a bleeding tendency, or a personal history of bruising or bleeding excessively, a detailed blood study and evaluation may be considered necessary. In some instances of mild bleeding tendencies, appropriate preoperative medications are recommended.

A history of allergic disorders must also be considered. Surgery of the nose cannot cure nasal allergies, although it can lessen breathing difficulties caused by an obstruction in the nasal passages. Allergies that are seasonal, such as hay fever and rose fever, do not contraindicate surgery, although the recovery period may be prolonged. Since rhinoplasty is an elective procedure, a time can be chosen for the operation when the offending pollens are not present in the air. There is a wide range of antihistamine preparations available which are generally helpful in making the allergic patient more comfortable. However, surgery can trigger latent allergies, and allergic patients should be aware that the operation could activate the symptoms.

On the positive side, allergies that are psychological or emotional in origin may improve after a successful rhinoplasty that has made the patients happy and feeling better about themselves.

No surgery should be performed in the presence of any respiratory infection.

One of the most important and sensitive aspects of an operation takes place at the first consultation between the patient and the surgeon. Whether or not there will be a good relationship between the surgeon and his prospective patient may depend upon what happens at this meeting. Psychological impressions will probably make the difference between acceptance or rejection of the surgeon by the potential patient—or the other way around. It is essential that the patient have a sense of complete confidence in the surgeon's ability and judgment, particularly since the final results of a rhinoplasty may not be apparent for months following the surgery and a patient with wavering faith in the doctor could experience some anguished moments.

First Consultation

And what about the surgeons? What are they looking for in a patient? Instant psychological analyses are not easy, nor are they always accurate, but experience and some poor decisions in the past in selecting patients have sharpened their intuitive sense about which patients are emotionally suited to the operation. Neuroses are as common as viruses these days, and doctors know from sad experience how neurotic, chronically dissatisfied patients can make life miserable for themselves, their families, and their surgeons, regardless of the finest aesthetic results.

At the first consultation, the surgeon finds out from the patient exactly what it is about the nose that is displeasing. After a physical examination, the surgeon will go into detail about what can be done and possible results in view of the patient's facial structure and skin; the inconveniences of the surgery; the appearance of the nose and face with the attendant swelling and discoloration following the removal of the bandages; and the period of convalescence. Patients whose physical conditions make them unlikely risks are discouraged from considering the surgery.

Among the patients who flash danger signals to the experienced surgeon are those whose concern with a minor nasal irregularity is out of all proportion to the defect; and patients whose concept of the outcome of the operation is totally inconsistent with what can reasonably be expected, or which the surgeon has described. It is difficult to deal with a patient whose self-image is divorced from reality. Surgeons know that rhinoplasty can do a great deal to bolster the ego of some people, but it can exacerbate the problems of those who have transferred their inner conflicts into a feeling of dissatisfaction with their noses. The latter is not uncommon and many of these people could profit by psychotherapy—not surgery. It is not always

79

easy to recognize the difference between the potential patient with a deep-rooted neurosis and the one whose concern is connected directly to a physical defect. Often the surgeon must rely on a sixth sense when deciding which patients are suitable candidates for surgery. Dr. R. tells the following story:

Clyde A., 28, a slim, sandy-haired young man, seemed very tense and nervous on his first visit to my office. He told me that he was an accountant, but he wanted to become an actor, and he felt that his appearance would militate against him. His nose was large and aquiline, with a sharply angled hump. His upper eyelids were crepey and hooded his eyes, and he had pouches underneath his eyes, which gave him a tired, dissipated look. He brought me a picture to give me an idea of what he wanted to look like. Altogether, he was practically a perfect textbook example of the kind of patient that plastic surgeons are warned against. But there was something about the young man that made me feel that his thinking and motivation were sound, even if his behavior suggested otherwise. I was torn between accepting him as a patient or recommending him to a psychiatrist, and purely on a hunch, I decided to do the former.

Anyway, he turned out to be a perfect patient. We had an excellent result and he was pleased and grateful. With the scaled-down nose and unwrinkled eyelids, he looked about 19 or 20. He called my office recently to say that he was auditioning for the juvenile lead in a play, but I don't know what happened. At any rate, if his acting career doesn't work out, he said he can always go back to being the most youthful-looking CPA in the business. But in the meantime he's doing what he wanted to do and it's a source of satisfaction for me to know I helped. By all odds, he was a most unlikely prospect ... it just shows how you never can be sure.

There is another element in the patient-doctor relationship when rhinoplasty is involved that is not present in other types of cosmetic surgery, except perhaps ear correction. It has to do with the age of the patients. The preponderance of patients being considered for surgery of the nose are young, many of them minors, which brings their families into the picture. In many cases, the young person sees the plastic surgeon under protest, literally dragged to the office by well-meaning but misguided parents. Surgeons have no trouble deciding about surgery in this kind of situation. They give first consideration to the wishes of the patient, regardless of parental pressure. They will discuss the operation and the results that may be expected, but they will refuse to operate until the young patients themselves wish it. Marjorie N. recalls her experience:

It took me a long time to forgive my mother for making me have a rhinoplasty. It was over 20 years ago and I still remember how furious I was. Of course my nose is all right, but I thought it was all right before the operation, too. It certainly never bothered me nor discouraged my boy friends, and having it done over was the last thing I wanted. But that was another era and I don't suppose it ever occurred to me to fight my family. But did I ever get even with them! I was an absolute demon for weeks after the operation, carrying on about the black and blue marks and not being able to smell or taste anything or breathe—actually, it was months before I could breathe easily.... I'm sure I made my poor mother sorry she ever started the whole thing.

But good intentions or not, it's wrong to push anybody into this kind of thing unless they want it themselves. I might have gotten around to thinking about my nose in a couple of years, but at that time it was a traumatic and unwelcome experience. I can just imagine how my 16-year-old would react if I suggested that she have her nose changed ... she'd wither me with a look.

Reluctant patients like Marjorie will inevitably have a stormier convalescence than the calm, cooperative patient who chose to have the operation for the right reasons. There is no doubt that the process of healing is influenced to a considerable degree by the patient's state of mind. The amount of trust and confidence the patient places in the surgeon will also have an effect on the postoperative course, and a good doctor-patient relationship can be most supportive for the patient.

But let it not be inferred that plastic surgeons are besieged by neurotic, emotionally unstable patients clamoring for unnecessary surgery. The majority of people who fill the waiting rooms of plastic surgeons are well-adjusted men and women with perfectly sound reasons for wishing to improve their appearance. They are people with no great emotional hang-ups; they just didn't happen to like the shape of the noses they were born with and decided to do something about it. But there are many instances where a complex human drama lies behind the need of the patient who seeks rhinoplasty.

The extent of the psychological damage that an unattractive nose can inflict on its wearer may elude those who have never had to deal with such a situation, but it is familiar to the plastic surgeon.

Lydia C., 60, is a first-rate commercial artist. She is an attractive woman with regular features that add up to a pleasing face. But it was not always so:

I think I was the unhappiest teenager in the world. My nose wasn't just bad—it was the quintessence of a beaked monstrosity. I was always small and thin, and that dreadful nose would have been too big for a six-foot-six-inch basketball player. At that time we were living in a small town in the Midwest and I don't ever recall hearing anything about plastic surgery. I was an only child—my father died when I was quite small—and my mother had a struggle to keep our modest household going, so even if there had been a plastic surgeon living next door, I don't think it would have done me any good. But in any event, my mother thought I was just about perfect. It was a good thing she liked me, because she saw a lot of me. On weekend nights when there were boy-girl parties, I stayed at home and drew pictures of pretty girls with small uptilted noses. As I look back, I realize that I was sharp-tongued and abrasive ... always on the defensive ... probably I was responsible for driving friends away—I'm not sure.

After I finished art school in New York, I started doing very well professionally. I did the art work for full-page advertisements in the Sunday Times *for some of the leading department stores, and all the drawings of the women had perfect noses on the small side. Talk about sublimation! There were no fine Roman noses on* my *ladies. When a magazine wanted to do a feature story about me with a photograph, I agreed—with the proviso that the picture show me holding a book that covered the lower half of my face and hid most of my nose.*

And then it dawned on me that I didn't have to live with that wretched nose. The minute I accumulated enough money, I made the rounds of plastic surgeons until I found Dr. H., to whom I'm everlastingly grateful. I remember my first visit to his office. I wanted so much to draw him a picture of the kind of nose I'd always dreamed of having, but I'd been told that plastic surgeons are usually doubtful about people who bring them pictures of noses they want copied, so I restrained myself. That was over 30 years ago and I haven't had to cover my face with a book to take a respectable picture ever since.

Actually, I've been more successful in my professional life than in my personal life. I've been married twice, and both times were disasters. Maybe I was partly to blame. I often wonder whether it might have been different if I'd been happier about myself while I was growing up ... but then, how am I ever going to know?

Before-and-After Photographs

The use of preoperative photographs can be particularly helpful to both patient and doctor in discussing rhinoplasty. With the photographs, the patients can pinpoint the changes they would like and the surgeons can indicate clearly what can and cannot be done and explain the reasons. This prepares the patients for the results and lessens the chances for disappointment and misunderstanding. Patients should understand, however, that they must rely on the judgment of the surgeon in determining the final size and shape of the nose, although any reasonable desires will always be considered by the surgeon.

Four views of the nose are taken: the two profiles, front face, and a view from under the nostrils.

The patient is admitted to the hospital the day before surgery. Routine physical examination of the patient and laboratory studies on blood and urine are performed. The night before surgery, the usual preoperative face cleansing is done using an antibacterial soap such as pHisoHex. Premedications are begun the night before surgery so that the patient will be calm and relaxed.

Some doctors recommend the use of antibiotics, begun 24 hours before surgery and continued for four days following. Because aspirin can promote bleeding, patients are advised not to take any before or after surgery.

Before
the Operation

Premedication is given several hours before surgery so that the patient is relaxed and drowsy before being taken to the operating room. The common experience among patients who have had rhinoplasty under local anesthesia is that they are aware of sounds and manipulation in their nasal region, but the memory of the operation—if indeed they do remember—is one without pain or tension.

Local anesthesia is usually used, although general anesthesia may be employed in highly apprehensive or younger patients, or if it is the choice of the surgeon. The services of an anesthesiologist are required when general anesthesia is used. The interior and exterior of the nose are injected with pain-killing drugs. There is no pain connected with these injections because of the previous medication. When the anesthesia is complete, the surgeon begins the operation.

Anesthesia

To remove a hump, part of bone and cartilage is removed (shaded area).

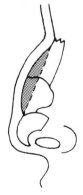

The surgery is performed entirely from inside the nose. The procedures for rhinoplasty may include removing the hump on the bridge of the nose or lowering the contour of a prominent

The Operation

83

nose (the dorsum); narrowing the nose to balance the flatness caused by the removal of the hump; shortening or lengthening the nose; and reshaping the tip. The sequence in which these steps are carried out varies. All plastic surgeons have their own approach to rhinoplasty and will choose the order of their procedures to suit the needs of the patient on whom they are operating. The correction of the septum can be combined with these procedures.

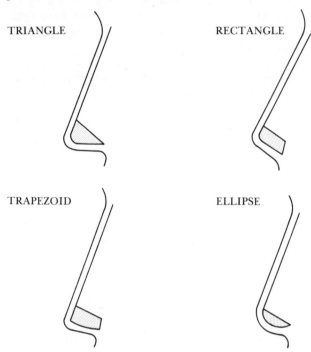

TRIANGLE

RECTANGLE

TRAPEZOID

ELLIPSE

Septal excisions in nasal corrections: a triangular excision tilts the nose tip, a rectangular excision shortens it, a trapezoidal one shortens and tilts, and an ellipse improves a hanging columella.

A scalpel is inserted between the skin and the bone in each nasal cavity to separate the skin from the underlying cartilage and bony framework. If the nose is to be shortened, the columella is also separated from the septum. To reshape the tip, the surgeon makes another incision within each nostril to expose the cartilages that form the tip and nostril rims. These cartilages are trimmed to obtain a graceful nose tip that will conform to the new profile. With a small surgical saw or chisel, the hump of the bridge is removed. The septum is cut shorter, or straightened, or lowered, according to the correction that is desired. A triangular excision of the septum tilts the tip of the nose; a rectangular excision shortens the nose; a trapezoidal incision both shortens and tilts; and an ellipse repairs a hanging columella. The nasal bones are then surgically fractured and molded into a new, slender position. It is the breaking of the nasal bones that is mainly responsible for the subsequent black and blue discoloration in and around the eyes and nose that every rhinoplasty patient is familiar with. Finally, the lining of the nose—the mucosa—is sutured.

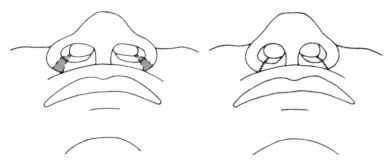

Flared nostrils are improved by removing a wedge. The scar is in an unnoticeable position in the crease of the nostril.

The skin over the bridge of the nose, being thin and elastic, will drape nicely over the new bony framework like a snug glove. However, lowering the height of the nose produces a slack in the wings or alae of the nose that may give the nostrils an unattractive flared look. This can be corrected by excising a wedge at the base of each nostril and closing the wound. The fine hairline scar is hidden in the crease of the nose where it curves to join the upper lip and is not conspicuous. On completion of the operation, the nose is generally lightly packed (some surgeons omit the packing) and a splint dressing is placed on the outside of the nose to hold down swellings and to protect the nose while it heals. The splints are held in place by strips of tape.

The operation may take from half an hour to an hour and a half, depending on the skill and experience of the surgeon and the complexity of the operation.

Nose Tip Correction

Plastic surgeons are frequently consulted about corrections only to the tip of the nose. It may have seemed to the potential patients that they brought about a great improvement in their appearance when they raised up the tip of their nose just the tiniest bit. However, an elongated tip is often part of an enlarged bone and the tip correction may involve more than appears at first glance. There are isolated situations where a tip correction would be indicated, as in the case of a previously performed rhinoplasty that required a secondary procedure, but more often, only complete rhinoplasty will yield a satisfactory result.

Patients contemplating such limited surgery should be guided by the advice of competent plastic surgeons whose experience with partial rhinoplasties has made them able to predict the results of such procedures.

Surgery of the tip is a comparatively simple operation. It does not involve fracturing the nasal bones, so consequently there would not be the usual discoloration that occurs with the total operation. The essential consideration is whether the results would justify the limited procedure.

Building Up the Nose

In contrast to the nose that nature has endowed too generously is the nose that is lacking in size or contour. A nose flattened or twisted by an accident or trauma; a nose with a depressed nasal bridge (saddle nose); a too-short nose with an exaggerated uptilt and large flared nostrils; and a nose that was overly modified by a previous rhinoplasty can be as objectionable to their owners as the too-large nose. Such noses need to be increased and built up. They present a challenge to the plastic surgeon, but one they are equipped to meet. They can restructure a profile using either grafts or implants. A graft, or transplant, is living tissue such as bone or cartilage taken from its original site—or from another person—and transferred to another part of the body. An implant is an inert substance (alloplastic), which is placed under the skin. Silicone compounds are the most popularly used implants at this time. Although many surgeons use the silicone implant to build up the desired contour of the nose, other surgeons prefer a graft of bone or cartilage. Each of these substances has its champions.

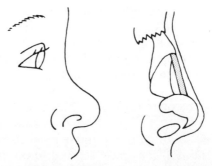

To correct a saddle nose, the depressed nasal bridge is built up by a cartilage implant (shaded area).

The surgeon carefully prepares the implant or graft on its undersurface to fit precisely where the bridge of the nose is depressed. The upper surface of the implant or graft will become the new contour of the nose. It is tailored to present the desired profile, straight or retroussé. The surgeon dissects a pocket high up in the nose straight along the depressed bridge, inserts the implant or the graft into the pocket, and closes the incision. The size of the pocket is carefully gauged so it will hold the implant or graft snugly in place.

If the tip of the nose also needs to be supported, as is often the case with the black African or Oriental nose, an L-shaped implant would be used. It is inserted through an incision in the columella or the lower part of the septum. The thin, elastic skin and mucosa that cover the upper part of the nose will have no difficulty in fitting easily over the new framework.

Variations and modifications of this technique are used in altering the black African and Oriental noses. The former is characterized by a flat, broad bridge with a rounded tip and flaring nostrils. In addition to elevating the bridge by an implant or graft and raising the tip, it is generally necessary to narrow the width of the nostrils by removing a wedge at the base of the nostrils, as described earlier. The surgeon may choose to use cartilage from the septum, when possible. Scarring and keloids are a danger in black skins, although some surgeons report that they have had no scarring complications in the wedge-removal procedure performed on black skins. Surgical discretion is always advisable, however, and patients should be made aware of the possibilities of scar formation.

The typical Oriental nose is small and accompanied by a slight recession of the upper lip. The most common rhinoplasties on Orientals involve elevating the nasal bridge by an implant or graft and reshaping the nostril rims and tip of the nose.

All plastic surgeons have their own procedures for the post-operative management of the rhinoplasty patient, which may differ somewhat from those of their colleagues. They are procedures that have worked for them and their patients and are suited to the particular techniques used during the surgery. Most surgeons, but not all, insert a light gauze packing inside the nose. A tight packing might be indicated where there was a badly deviated septum and an extensive resection was done. However, a splint is always applied to the outside of the nose to help prevent bleeding, to hold down swelling, and to protect the nose. The splint is held in place with strips of adhesive tape. Some doctors use a pressure dressing and ice compresses over the eyes for a number of hours after the operation to inhibit swelling and discoloration.

The packing in the nose may be removed anywhere from 24 to 48 hours or longer following the surgery, depending on the judgment of the surgeon. When extensive reconstruction has been done on the septum to correct a crooked nose, the packing

Completing the Operation

may be left in for from three to five days. The time that the splints are retained likewise varies. Some surgeons remove them after three or four days, whereas others leave them in place for seven to ten days, on the premise that the patient has a sense of security from knowing that the new nose is protected.

There is a slight, bloody discharge from the nose following the operation that gradually decreases in a day or two. After the nasal packing is removed, there can be some stuffiness of the nose caused by swelling and the accumulation of crusts. The surgeon recommends appropriate measures that provide some relief for this problem.

Sometimes the nasal bones spread a bit after the splint is taken off, resulting in the widening of the upper nose. The surgeon may be able to correct this by pressing the bones together once or twice a week for a number of weeks. This can be painful, but it is frequently effective.

The usual hospital stay for a rhinoplasty is from one or two days to four or five days, depending on the patient, the surgeon, and the circumstances.

Patients are generally not in any pain immediately following surgery; the discomfort they experience comes from the packing in the nose and the resulting difficulty in breathing. The chief complaint is generally the dry throat that comes from having to breathe through the mouth. Most patients have black and blue discoloration in and around the eyes and a swollen lip and nose tip. As a rule, the patients look much worse than they feel.

The Splint Comes Off

Patients are always warned that the final results of the rhinoplasty will not be evident immediately. Unlike other facial cosmetic operations in which the improvements are apparent within days, the nose may not assume its final shape for weeks or even months. The patient must be prepared for less than a vision of loveliness when the splint is removed. The nose and eyes may still be discolored and swollen. A snub-nosed look is not uncommon, because the surgeon often overcorrects the tip in an upward position, knowing that it will drop somewhat from the effects of gravity and relaxation of the scar tissue. It is quite different from presenting a finished sculpture that the artist has smoothed and burnished to its ultimate degree of perfection. The surgeon has constructed the foundation and framework, and now the healing processes will take over. Many patients are understandably apprehensive about the "unveiling" of the nose. Jenny S. described her experience:

The nose splint was coming off the next day, but that night I had a terrible nightmare: when Dr. J. removed the splint, my face would come

88

with it—there would be nothing left but a formless blob. "Ready?" Dr. J. said.

He took the splint off. No trumpets, except in my head. My naked face smiled at me in the mirror. It was swollen and distorted. Pinkish bruises framed my nose, but no purple. Nothing fell off. The nose itself looked like a boiled potato.

In just a few days, the major swelling would disappear, the doctor said. (It did.) Then, gradually, over two to three months, the final nose would take shape. (It did.) At this point, the nose looked short and squashy but, he assured me, it would "drop".... My nose felt tender to the touch.

Caring for the New Nose

Once the new nose has healed completely, it will be as substantial as it ever was, needing no more thought or pampering than before. But for the first few weeks immediately after the operation, certain precautions must be taken. The bones of the nose knit slowly and can be easily disturbed during that time.

The nose must not be blown for ten days following surgery, and then most gently for the next several weeks. For the first few days following the operation, it can be mopped lightly on the outside with a tissue. After the packing is removed, the nostrils can be lightly cleaned with a cotton-tipped applicator dipped in a bland ointment. The surgical trauma causes congestion in the mucous membranes and as a result, the nose often feels stuffy, like a minor head cold. However, this generally clears within the first month.

Eyeglasses may generally be worn after the splint is removed, although they may leave a temporary dent in the swollen skin at the bridge. There is a way of keeping the glasses off the bridge of the nose by suspending them from the forehead with a strip of Scotch tape wound around the nosepiece of the glasses. Contact lenses may be inserted immediately.

For the first week after surgery, patients should avoid places that are excessively air conditioned, such as restaurants and movies. Strenuous physical activities should be limited for three weeks, but this does not mean that patients should invalid themselves. Generally patients can return to their regular routine of school or work in about a week if they are comfortable about the way they look and if the work is fairly sedentary and not physically demanding. After the third week, the patient can swim in calm water—no ocean bathing or diving—or play tennis or golf. They should not consider playing any body contact sport such as football, soccer, or wrestling for four to six months following a rhinoplasty. For the first two or three weeks, any other body contact activity that might involve the nose, such as kissing, should be engaged in with restraint.

Hair washing is generally postponed for ten days to two

weeks. The heat of the dryer should be directed away from the nose, as much as possible. Exposure to the sun is to be assiduously avoided for three weeks, and then only moderate exposure is permitted. Sunburn with its accompanying swelling, redness, and peeling is highly undesirable.

Patients should not palpate the nose unnecessarily, unless expressly ordered by the surgeon. Sometimes surgeons suggest that the patient press the nasal bones together periodically to compress them.

It is also advisable during cold weather, when houses are heated artificially, to add moisture to the air. This can be done by placing a pan of water on the radiator or using a humidifier. The moisture in the air helps to prevent the mucous membranes in the nose from drying out during the night and forming small encrustations that may separate and bleed.

Most people are fairly presentable after about a week, and within two or three weeks healing is well started and the patient begins to feel more at home with the new nose.

Complications   Serious and prolonged complications after rhinoplasty are rare. Aside from the minor problems of swelling and nasal congestion that may persist, the most common complication of rhinoplasty is postoperative bleeding. It can occur at any time from immediately following surgery to 10 to 14 days later. It can be serious enough to require the patient to reenter the hospital. When it occurs within the first 48 hours, the packing is removed from the nose and fresh packing containing medication that controls bleeding is gently inserted. In most instances, careful packing with medicated gauze will control the bleeding, but when the hemorrhage is quite severe, special treatment may be required. Fortunately, this type of hemorrhage happens rarely, but surgeons are ever aware of the possibility of this complication.

Infection following rhinoplasty is most unusual and the antibiotics that most surgeons prescribe before and after surgery provide further protection. The sense of numbness in the nose that is usually experienced is temporary and passes quickly.

A diminished sense of smell (with the accompanying lessening of the sense of taste) may follow rhinoplasty, but this generally corrects itself in a few weeks. In a small percentage of cases, however, it may continue for up to a year. It would be most unusual for rhinoplasty to cause protracted or permanent damage to the sense of smell. It is more common to find that the correction of a deviated septum is beneficial to the sense of smell.

Sometimes there are minor skin complications from sensitivity to the tapes that hold the dressings and splints in place. These irritations generally respond well to a wide selection of cortisone creams and there are also hypo-allergenic tapes that are tolerated by most skins.

When there is an unsatisfactory result because of inept surgery, an injury before healing is completed, or a quirk in the patient's healing ability, a secondary procedure can be performed with good results if there is sufficient cartilage, bony framework, and tissue to work with. Certain damages can be repaired, but it is generally more difficult to achieve a first-rate aesthetic result in succeeding rhinoplasties than in the first.

Follow-Up Visits

The frequency of postoperative visits to the doctor's office following rhinoplasty varies with each surgeon. After the packing and splint removal, surgeons generally see patients once a week for the first month, then every other week, gradually tapering off with longer intervals between visits as the healing progresses satisfactorily. The doctor may see the patient for up to a year following the operation. The patient is asked to return for the "after" photographs when the doctor thinks the nose has assumed its permanent shape.

There is no charge for follow-up visits.

Fees

Fees for rhinoplasty vary according to the experience of the surgeon, the area of the country, and the complexity of the operation. The fee range is from $500 to $2,000 and upwards. An average fee would probably be in the neighborhood of $1,500. If a revision or a secondary procedure is necessary, surgeons perform them on their own patients without an additional fee.

Medical insurance does not cover a rhinoplasty performed for purely cosmetic reasons, but if a medical condition such as a deviated septum requires correction, part of the surgeon's fee and the anesthesiologist's, if general anesthesia is given, is reimbursed.

The Afterglow

The majority of patients who have had rhinoplasties are satisfied and enthusiastic. Often the operation has a more profound effect than only a change in appearance. Many people find themselves recharged with a surge of self-confidence and self-esteem. Women particularly become more concerned with their total look and take a fresh interest in their clothes, figures, and general grooming. Nora M.'s experience illuminates this. Nora is a young, good-looking, 38-year-old sports clothes designer. Her straight, well-proportioned nose is the result of a rhinoplasty performed six months earlier.

There have been so many changes in my life in the last six months, and I'm sure none of them would have happened if I hadn't had the rhino-plasty. The whole thing started almost a year ago with a new hair style. It was a great hairdo, but it was all wrong with my nose. My nose was too long and too pointed and there was a hump on the bridge. I thought it was horrendous. I always hated it. A friend recommended a plastic surgeon who had just done her nose—it was beautiful—and I decided the time had come.

The operation went well and according to schedule. Everything the surgeon had told me would happen did. I was completely relaxed during the operation and felt no pain ... there was a curious sense of detach-ment. I heard the sounds of cracking bone and sawing and grinding— but it was all as if it were happening to somebody else and I was perched somewhere in the operating room looking on. The operation might have been a little more involved than some because I had a deviated septum that had to be corrected. There was no pain after the operation—just discomfort from having to breathe through my mouth.

My convalescence was equally uneventful. I had the usual bloodshot eyes and lots of black and blue and considerable swelling, but after the fourth or fifth day there was a noticeable improvement as each day passed. I went back to work two weeks after the operation but it took about three weeks until all the discoloration had disappeared. My breathing was slightly constricted for the next few months, but that finally cleared. I played tennis a month after the surgery.

The new nose and the new hairdo, which finally went together, started me on a self-improvement kick, and I got around to shedding the five pounds that I'd been meaning to get rid of for a long time. But that was just the beginning.

I'd been unhappy in my job for years and I could never bring myself to do anything about it. I consider myself reasonably creative and the scope of my work was so limited that it was stifling whatever talent I have in that direction. But I think my new look gave me the courage to resign and look for something else. It was one of the best things I've ever done . . . . I was offered a new job that gives me the opportunity for the imaginative, original work that I had been missing. I feel as if I have a whole new lease on life—I feel so much better about myself and what I am capable of.

I'm sorry I didn't have the rhinoplasty years ago. When I think of the time and energy I used up hating my nose and being unhappy over it—and now I never have to think about it anymore. It's as if I were relieved of an uncomfortable burden.

Most people have a rhinoplasty because they are dissatisfied with the appearance of their nose and want it improved. Joan T.'s reason was refreshingly different and unique—but then, not everyone is married to a plastic surgeon.

Joan and David were high-school sweethearts who married while David was still in medical school. By that time, Joan had graduated from college and was on the way to a successful career in the fashion world. Joan was a dynamic, chic, highly attractive young woman, in spite of a nose not dissimilar to the "before" section of the "before-and-after" photographs of rhinoplasties. The nose had a hump and a curve and an overhanging tip—surely an imperfect nose, but one that was in complete harmony with a pleasing and distinctive face. It never occurred to anyone to comment that she would be good-looking if her nose were different. She *was* good-looking.

In due course, David finished medical school, his internship, his residency, and finally he took off on what turned out to be a distinguished career in plastic surgery.

Shortly after David opened his first office, he and Joan were at the theater and found themselves seated next to a patient on whom David had recently performed a rhinoplasty. During intermission, introductions were exchanged and the patient was effusive in praise of her surgeon and her new nose. Joan, not yet quite at home in the role of the surgeon's wife, felt constrained to make some appropriate comment.

"It's lovely," she said. "I've been looking at your nose."

"Yes," said the patient, "and I've been looking at yours."

Of course you can guess what happened next. And did Joan's life change with her new nose? Not at all. But it hadn't needed to. Joan became prettier, but not necessarily any better-looking. Her new hair style with bangs would have been an impossibility with the former nose. Her face took on a softness and piquancy that it had not had before but it perhaps lost a bit of its distinctiveness along the way. However, Joan was safe from censure from her husband's patients.

NASAL
RECONSTRUCTION

Before

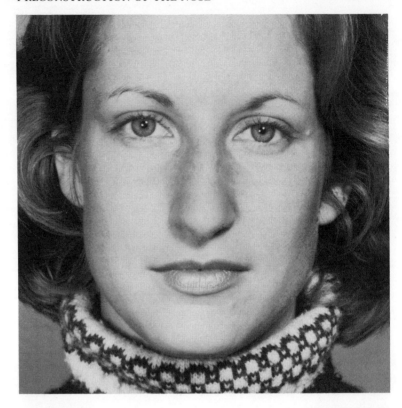

After

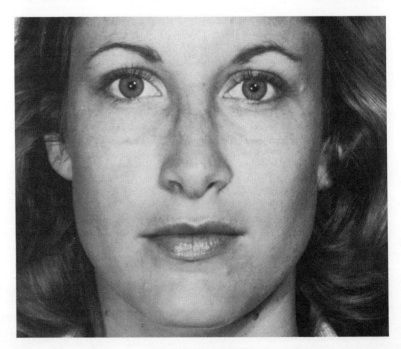

Before

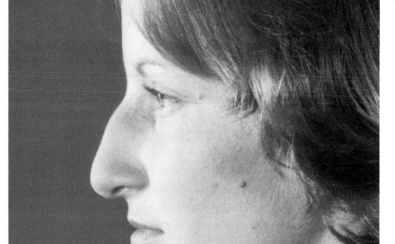

After

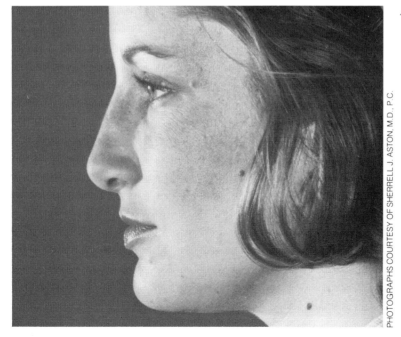

PHOTOGRAPHS COURTESY OF SHERRELL J. ASTON, M.D., P.C.

**NASAL
RECONSTRUCTION**
Before

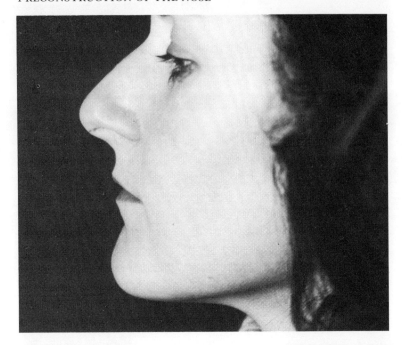

After

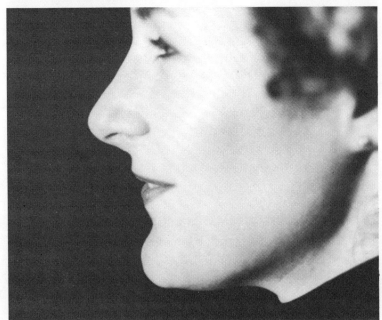

PHOTOGRAPHS COURTESY OF THE PATIENT

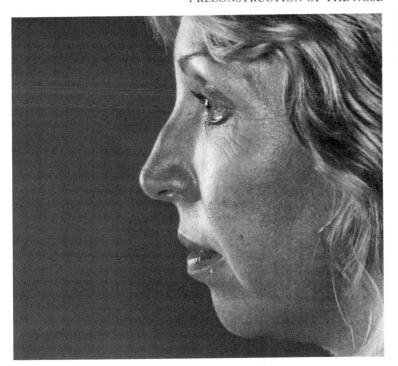

NASAL
RECONSTRUCTION
AND CHIN IMPLANT
Before

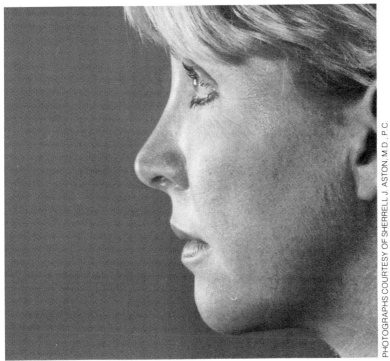

After

PHOTOGRAPHS COURTESY OF SHERRELL J. ASTON, M.D., P.C.

97

5

Jaw, Chin, and Lip Correction

A jaw or chin that is too large, too small, or poorly constructed can detract from the balance and harmony of the human face. It can also convey a misleading impression about its owner. While there is no proof that the shape of a chin has anything to do with a person's character, people are often stereotyped as weak or timid, stubborn or belligerent because of a genetic or developmental accident that carved out the shape of the lowest third of their faces. Plastic surgery can correct many of the errors made when nature becomes too lavish or too stingy and produces an overdeveloped or underdeveloped jaw or chin.

The quest for surgery of the chin and jaw often goes beyond a desire for aesthetic improvement. Faulty relationship between the jaws caused by too much or too little growth in one or both of the jaws may interfere with proper chewing, breathing, or speaking. Jaws and teeth can be so formed that the lips will not close over the teeth without straining. In situations such as these, the problem takes on the added dimension of functional impairment and looks to oral surgery for help.

The last decade has witnessed the most dramatic advances in orthognathic or orthodontic surgery. This is surgery for the correction of irregularities of the jaw that result in dental and facial deformities. Procedures that were once rarely done, such as cutting the maxilla (upper jaw), are now routinely performed. Almost any portion of either jawbone, the maxilla or the mandible (lower jaw), can be cut and moved in any direction required to achieve the objectives of good looks and proper bite. Sections of jawbone and teeth can be excised and the jaw restructured and reshaped when necessary. Jaw defects that not so long ago were the despair of plastic and oral surgeons can now be corrected.

Orthognathic surgery is not restricted to one medical or dental discipline. It is performed by plastic surgeons and oral surgeons. While plastic surgery is essentially concerned with soft tissues, it also encompasses certain corrections to the bony structure of the jaws. The oral surgeon has had specialized training in this area and often the correction of a complex jaw deformity requires the services of a team consisting of the plastic surgeon, the oral surgeon, and the orthodontist. The orthodontist is a dentist who specializes in the proper positioning and relationship of the teeth.

Major Jaw Surgery 　Generally the upper and lower jaws grow at about the same rate so that when they reach adult size, the teeth meet properly, the tongue and lips rest in a comfortable position, and the contour of the face is harmonious and pleasing. But nature sometimes becomes capricious, and for no known reason, one or the other of the jaws may stop growing before it reaches maturity or it becomes overdeveloped, disrupting the balance of the face and the health of the teeth and gums. When dentistry and orthodontia cannot help, corrective bone surgery to improve the skeletal framework is called for. Extraordinary results are achieved in improving overlong chins that add excessive facial height, in bringing symmetry to jaws completely lacking it, in restoring chins so recessive they barely exist, and in aligning jaws so poorly positioned that both the meshing of the teeth and the appearance of the face are adversely affected. Most of the operations are now performed from inside the mouth with no visible scars left behind as a reminder.

Many of the techniques now in use were developed after World War II as a means of repairing the facial structure of men disfigured by battle injuries. Jaws that were broken in two, three, or more places were restored successfully. The oral surgeons reasoned that if these reconstructive procedures worked for injuries, they might also be applied on an elective basis to correct jaw deformities. Why could the jaws not be broken if necessary, and repositioned to correct the functional or aesthetic impairment of the teeth, jaws, and contour of the face? And so the lessons learned from injuries were directed toward elective surgery to the advantage of people who had never dared to hope it was possible to look more attractive.

The Development of Oral Surgery 　Oral surgery is not a new art, but it is a comparatively new specialty. In the 19th Century, complicated operations on the mouth and jaw were performed by general surgeons since there were no oral surgeons and many of the techniques used at that time are still valid today. The operations were performed only when the patient's life or health were threatened; surgery to improve the appearance had not yet entered the scene. When, in 1893, President Grover Cleveland was discovered to have cancer of the upper jaw, the operation to remove it was performed by one of the leading general surgeons of that time. The entire left upper jaw was removed and replaced by an artificial jaw made of vulcanized rubber. The operation was a complete success and there was no recurrence.

The turn of the century saw bold and innovative work being done and oral surgery was developing into a specialty. One of the earliest organizations of oral surgeons, the American Association of Oral and Plastic Surgeons, was formed in 1918. It was followed in 1921 by the formation of an organization called the American Society of Oral Surgery and Exodontia, which in 1943 became the American Society of Oral Surgeons. The American Board of Oral Surgeons came into being in April 1947. This is the prestigious organization that certifies oral specialists. Today many major hospitals in large cities throughout the United States have instituted residency programs in oral surgery that turn out highly trained specialists.

Candidates for Jaw Surgery

Most of the patients who elect to have extensive jaw surgery are in their teens or their twenties. Except for the repair of a cleft palate, surgery should not generally be performed on the jaws until they have reached their full growth. If done earlier, there is the possibility of a relapse as the patient's jaws continue to grow. Some surgeons feel that 16 is the minimum age. Such surgery is not necessarily contraindicated for older persons, although they may not be as good candidates for the complex procedures sometimes necessary to change the contour of the jaw and improve the bite. Nevertheless, people in their fifties have been operated on successfully. But more often, the older person has become accustomed to living with the condition and may be reluctant to undergo the inconveniences of the surgery. Chin and jaw improvement for the mature patient is more likely to be limited to a chin implant, which will be discussed later in this chapter.

Planning Major Oral Surgery

The oral surgeon and orthodontist spend hours of planning and research in preparation for major oral surgery. Each step of the operation is known and planned in advance, from the exact position of the first incision to the smallest detail of how many millimeters of bone are to be removed.

To accomplish this, the surgeon works with the patient's life-size medical photographs of both profiles, cephalograms, dental casts of the jaws and teeth, a set of dental films, and a model of the patient's bite. The cephalogram is a special x-ray of the skull in profile that shows the relationship of the teeth to the skeleton and the soft tissue.

The cephalometric x-ray was first developed by orthodontists who have a special interest in the balance between the teeth,

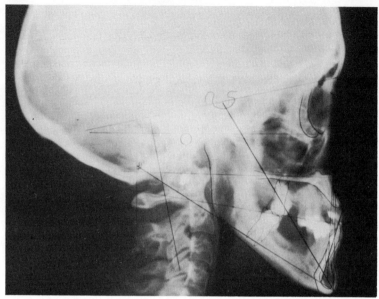

Lines and angles drawn on cephalometric x-ray indicate to the oral surgeon the nature and degree of the patient's jawbone defect.

bony framework, and skin covering of the lower face. A head holder with short earposts that enter the patient's ear is used to take the cephalometric x-ray. The source of radiation is lined up with the earposts. Since this arrangement places the patient's head in a fixed position, it is possible to take preoperative and postoperative x-rays from exactly the same angle. This is helpful in evaluating the surgical or orthodontic changes that occur.

The cephalogram is a most valuable diagnostic tool. On a transparent sheet of acetate placed over the cephalogram, the surgeon draws lines to and from a number of fixed points of reference that reveal such information as the exact length of certain bones, the relationship of the jaws to the face and to each other, and the relationship of the teeth to the jaw. Based on anthropological studies, the length of the lines and the width of the angles will indicate to some degree the extent of the patient's jawbone defect. The surgeon can determine, for instance, if the lower jaw is too big or if it appears that way because the upper jaw is too small and not in the correct position.

It is interesting to note that over the years attempts have been made to work out a precise mathematical formula for the proportions of a beautiful face, but there were always too many variables among beautiful faces to establish any firm conclusions. This was substantiated by cephalometric research on women of outstanding loveliness, such as models, film actresses, and beauty contest winners. The cephalograms on these women confirmed the fact that the dimensions, angles, and balance of the bones and soft tissues of their faces fitted within the broad ranges previously established, but again, there were many variables. It would be helpful in diagnosis and treatment planning if the proportions of a beautiful face could be translated into a clear-cut formula, but obviously the subtleties in the relationships of bony structure and covering skin are too elusive to be contained in a set of specific measurements. Perhaps that was what the 18th-Century English poet Alexander Pope meant when he wrote, "'Tis not a lip, or eye we beauty call/But the joint force and full result of all." It appears to be the "joint force" that defies capture by a mathematical formula.

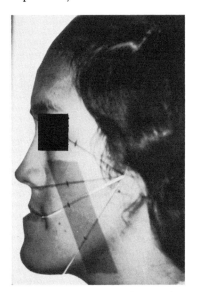 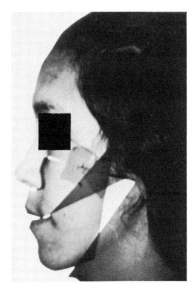

Profile photograph (left) is cut into segments and rearranged (right). Compare rearranged picture with actual final photograph on page 121.

In the preoperative planning of the operation, the oral surgeon duplicates the dental casts. At least three sets—sometimes more—are needed, for there is always more than one way to solve a problem. The surgeon works with the casts, juggling them into position until the proper meshing of teeth is achieved. The life-size profile photographs are particularly helpful in evaluating the balance between the nose and the chin and in determining where and how much change is needed. The photographs are cut into segments representing the planes of the face. The surgeon moves and shifts these segments like a jigsaw puzzle until the desired profile is achieved. The final placement of the sections will be a reasonably accurate representation of the profile after surgery.

103

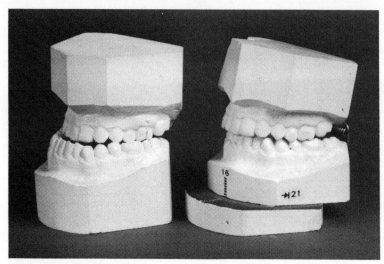

Plaster molds show prognathic jaw before and after surgery for repositioning of lower jaw.

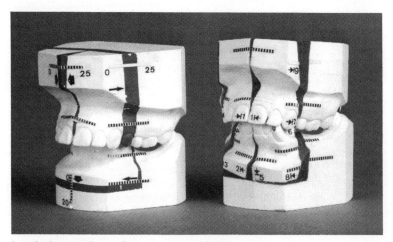

Surgical procedures for correction of protruding upper jaw are marked on study molds.

Every step of the operation is first carried out on the study model. In this respect, oral surgery is different from surgery on other parts of the body. In abdominal surgery, for example, the surgeons match their maneuvers to the conditions of tissues and organs they find as they proceed. But in orthodontic surgery, the surgeon knows in advance exactly how much bone is to be cut, what section of the jawbone is to be moved and how much, and what teeth must be sacrificed, or moved, or ground down. The surgeon charts the course of the operation according to the complicated and precise calculations made in the preliminary

104

study. The measurements derived from the cephalometric tracings are tested on the dental study molds. There is no margin for error in oral surgery and the entire surgical procedure planned for the patient is first performed on the study molds.

The oral surgeon makes every effort not to sacrifice any teeth, but it may be unavoidable if the new position of the jaws requires it. Tooth adjustments after jaw surgery are not unusual, but by careful planning in advance, the surgeon tries to avoid unnecessary loss of tooth structure.

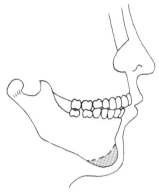

Slightly protruding lower jaw may be treated by scraping or filing excess bone (shaded area).

The correction of a protruding jaw—prognathia—is a major surgical procedure. Prognathia is an enlargement of the lower jaw in which the jaw juts forward. True prognathism is always accompanied by malocclusion (failure of the upper and lower teeth to meet properly). The lower teeth are forward of the corresponding upper teeth. The purpose of the operation is to reposition the lower jaw so that the teeth will meet properly and the contour of the face will be improved. The techniques used in the operation will be determined largely by the extent of the malocclusion and the amount of repositioning of the lower jaw that is necessary.

Occasionally the protrusion of the lower jaw is slight and the teeth meet properly. This is not true prognathism. The excess bony growth of the chin can be reduced by filing or scraping with a suitable instrument. The operation may be performed either through an incision under the chin (submental), which leaves a small scar, or through the inside of the mouth (intraoral), which leaves no external scar. However, some surgeons report that the results of this procedure are often disappointing because the soft tissue of the chin pad is slightly affected, if at all, by the excision of bone, and the contour of the chin may not be enough improved to justify the procedure.

Correcting the Protruding Jaw

As a preliminary step to the surgical correction of a true prognathic jaw, the patient's teeth and gums should be in the best possible condition, with all decayed teeth and gum disease properly treated. If orthodontia is indicated, it should be done prior to surgery. However, in certain cases, postoperative orthodontia is recommended.

The Operation for
Protruding Jaw

The patient is generally admitted to the hospital the day before the operation. A complete physical examination, chest x-rays, and laboratory tests are done to make sure the patient is in good health. Special orthodontic appliances are placed in the mouth before surgery. These are used to hold the wires that immobilize the jaws during the healing period. Usually four to six weeks or longer are required for sufficient healing to occur before the jaws are allowed to move. The exact length of time depends on the patient's general health and the extent of the surgery.

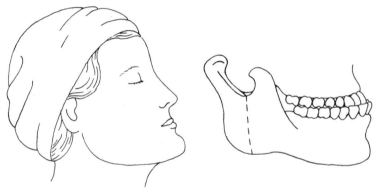

To correct a protruding lower jaw, or prognathia, the jawbone is cut on both sides (dashed line).

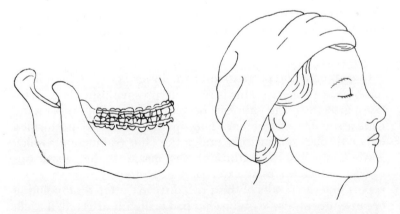

Lower jaw is slid back and teeth wired together to hold jaws in place. The result has jaws in proper position to each other.

106

The operation is performed under general anesthesia. The surgery may be done from the outside or entirely from inside the mouth, depending upon the amount of jaw protrusion, the position of the teeth, and the judgment of the surgeon. There are a number of different techniques employed in the correction of prognathia. In one procedure, a small incision is made in the natural neck crease below the angle of the jaw. The incision is carried upward to expose the lower border and angle of the mandible (lower jaw) and the bone is cut with an oscillating saw aided by an air drill. This is repeated on the opposite side of the jaw and the mandible is slid backward. The wounds are closed with fine sutures. After the jaw is brought to its new position, it is stabilized to the jaw by rubber bands, and the teeth are wired together to hold the jawbones securely in the correct position until healing is complete. The operation may take from two to four hours, depending on the complexity of the surgery.

After the Operation

This is a debilitating operation and the patient may feel quite weak after regaining consciousness, but the majority of patients are not excessively uncomfortable. A firm elastic pressure bandage is kept on the face for 48 hours to hold down the swelling. Medication for pain may be needed for a few days, but the pain will diminish as time passes. For the first few days following surgery, the patient is given medication, vitamins, and nourishment intravenously.

There is considerable swelling of the face for the first few days, but this will quickly lessen. The average hospital stay is about a week, and another week at home is required for convalescence. For the period of time that the jaws are wired together, the patient is limited to a liquid diet, generally sipped through a straw. This may not be quite as grim as it sounds, for all manner of foods, such as meats, fruits, and vegetables, can be liquefied in a blender. The net results may not be as inspiring as, say, a Maine lobster with drawn butter, but they can be tasty, varied, and nourishing. Even though the jaws are wired together, the patient is able to speak. An actor or actress might have to take a leave of absence from work, but the average business or professional person will be able to communicate satisfactorily. There may be numbness in the mouth that lasts for weeks or even months but it gradually passes.

Follow-Up

The patient is examined at least twice a week for the first two weeks following surgery, then once a week until the appliances are removed. Some oral surgeons schedule postoperative visits at longer intervals for the next six months and at six-month intervals for three years following surgery.

Fees

The oral surgeon's fee ranges from $1,500 to $5,000, depending upon the type of surgery, the area of the country, and the experience of the surgeon. Postoperative care is included in the fee. The fee for preoperative evaluation of the patient's jaw and mouth ranges from $150 to $200. It includes x-rays, cephalometric x-rays, dental study molds, and profile photographs. The orthodontist's fee ranges from $1,500 to $2,500.

Often hospital costs for functional jaw repair (as differentiated from purely cosmetic procedures) are covered by insurance. The amount of coverage depends on the patient's policy and should be discussed with the insurance carrier and not with the surgeon. The anesthetist's fee varies, depending on the nature of the operation, and it may also be covered by insurance.

A Patient's Experience

The surgical procedure to correct a prognathic jaw is a formidable operation, as Sandy B. will attest. Sandy's jaw was operated on six months earlier, and her memory of the experience is still vivid. Sandy is a pretty, vivacious young woman who looks younger than her 28 years. She is married and has a 2½-year-old child. A softly curved mouth, well-formed chin, pert nose, and expertly made-up large brown eyes are becomingly framed by swirling shoulder-length blond hair. It is difficult to imagine that just half a year ago, Sandy's face had a completely different contour and expression. An overdeveloped jaw jutted forward, giving her face a hard look. The lips met, but the lower lip bulged and was disproportionately large in relation to the upper lip. She had typical prognathic malocclusion with the lower teeth projecting beyond the top teeth.

"No, I don't suppose anyone thought of me as having a deformity—it wasn't as bad as that," Sandy replied in answer to the question. "But I always felt unattractive ... always. Ever since I was a teenager I've been self-conscious about my jaw and teeth, but I tried to cope with it. I never wore lipstick because I didn't want to call attention to my mouth. I rarely smiled because it made my jaw jut forward even more. I trained myself to smile with my mouth closed." She smiled a wide, spontaneous, uninhibited smile exposing two rows of even white teeth.

If Sandy was so unhappy about her jaw, why hadn't she attended to it before?

"Because I'm a marshmallow where pain is concerned," she said. "I suppose you could say I have a very low threshold for pain. My own dentist discouraged me about the operation, perhaps because he knew how I reacted to pain.

108

"It took a chain reaction—a series of events to get me to the point where I was ready to take on the operation. My first serious encounter with pain was the birth of my son. I had a very long difficult labor, but it finally came to an end—and I survived it. That was one up for the marshmallow. Then I had an accident on the tennis court and my nose was bashed in. It had to be operated on and I survived that. By that time I decided that maybe I wasn't really such a marshmallow.

"The plastic surgeon who repaired my nose encouraged me to have my jaw corrected. He referred me to an oral surgeon and that was when the idea really took off. The baby and the nose were—well, not exactly acts of God, but they weren't quite elective either. The jaw, though—that was something I wanted to do for myself."

Sandy described her meeting with the oral surgeon. Based on his clinical examination, he told her what could be done and what would be entailed. Her jaws would have to be immobilized for about eight weeks. He explained that he would do the operation from inside the mouth and there would be no scars, and he showed her preoperative and postoperative photographs of patients with conditions similar to hers.

Sandy would have been agreeable to going into the hospital the next day, but the preparation for oral surgery cannot be hurried. About six weeks were needed, for there were the preliminary studies involving x-rays, cephalograms, plaster casts of her jaws and teeth, and other tests to be completed and evaluated. Sandy had three impacted wisdom teeth that had to be removed and the gums given time to heal. Later on, the surgeon gave Sandy a preview of her new profile, using her life-size profile photographs, which had been cut into sections and rearranged.

"And that's exactly how it looked on the cut up photograph." She turned her head and exhibited a very nice profile.

"My surgeon does something else that's helpful. He has his prospective patients talk to other patients who have had the operation and it's most encouraging. Except..." She hesitated. "They all mentioned discomfort after the operation but nobody said anything about pain. I don't think the two words are synonymous and what I felt after surgery was *not* discomfort. But maybe that's my low threshold again."

Sandy encountered some strange reactions among her friends at the news of her plans for surgery. Her husband and family were most supportive but a few of her friends wondered whether she was harboring some secret plans for her future. A new career? A new man in her life? Otherwise, why would she be considering such a demanding operation—one that she could conceivably live without? "What nonsense," said Sandy. "As if I didn't have a divine child and the nicest, handsomest husband in the world." Quite properly, she ignored the innuendos.

The scheduled date for admission to the hospital finally arrived. The usual preoperative tests and examinations were completed and a specially fitted metal appliance was placed on her teeth. Already anxious and depressed, this upset her even more.

"It was horrendous," said Sandy. "A great heavy metal thing that I was sure would be intolerable. The surgeon said I'd get used to it after a while and I suppose I did, since it stayed in my mouth for the whole eight weeks that my jaws were wired closed and I lived with it. There were moments the day before the operation that I wondered if I hadn't made a great mistake, but I managed to put that thought behind me."

Finally came the big sleep of unconsciousness during the four hours of surgery and the awakening to find her face encased in an uncomfortable heavy elastic bandage placed there to inhibit the swelling. The bandage was removed after 48 hours. The next day or two passed in a blur of misery with intravenous feeding and medication, numbness, pain, a tremendously swollen face, and sticky hair. The swelling reached its peak in two or three days and then slowly began to lessen.

Sandy was out of bed in a few days. Ice cream sucked from a spoon became a favorite food. She returned home after about a week in the hospital. By the third week after the operation, Sandy was shopping, going to movies, and seeing her friends. Her lower face and lips were still swollen a bit. "I looked like a chipmunk," she said, but each day saw an improvement. Her wired jaw did not keep her from playing tennis and she had no difficulty in speaking or being understood even through the clenched jaws.

Eight weeks after the surgery the wires were removed. It took a day or two before she could open and close her jaws normally and a week before she could chew with ease and comfort.

"When the wires came off, I felt like a new person—as if I'd been born again.

"Was it worth it? Would I recommend the operation to other people who have the same condition as I had? While I was in the hospital, I would have said no. But my answer now is a decided yes. I'm happy with the way I look. My bite is the way it ought to be and even my speech is better. Before, my tongue rested on my lower teeth and I had a kind of whistling S sound that I couldn't do anything about. It was a 'tonguey' speech.

"I found the operation an ordeal—perhaps others might not find it as trying as I did—but it's one of the most rewarding things I've ever done."

There are a number of other conditions in which poor relationships of the jaws to each other, malocclusion, and lack of facial harmony require bone cutting (osteotomy) of the lower jaw (mandible). Among them are conditions known as micrognathia and retrognathia. They are less common than prognathia. Micrognathia is characterized by an underdeveloped, recessive chin with severe malocclusion. Retrognathia is a condition in which the lower jaw is normal in size but the chin is receded and there is mild malocclusion. Various operative techniques are used to correct these conditions. The corrections in both conditions require bone cutting and repositioning of the jaws, with immobilization of the jaws by wiring the teeth together until healing is complete.

Other Kinds of Major Jaw Surgery

Some jaw surgery involves moving only a part of the jaw. The operations to move the upper front segment of the jaw to correct buckteeth, or to reduce facial height by shortening the height of the mandible by removing a wedge of bone from it are examples. Procedures such as these do not usually require fastening the jaws shut.

A second category of corrective jaw surgery is the treatment of a minor structural defect known as microgenia, "small chin," which can usually be remedied by the insertion of an implant. An implant is an artificial material buried beneath the skin, in contradistinction to a graft or transplant which is a fragment of bone or cartilage taken from its original site and transferred to another part of the body. The implant builds out the chin, increasing its size. This procedure is called chin augmentation, or, to give it its medical name, mentoplasty augmentation. Most of the operations performed on the chin by plastic surgeons are for this condition.

Correcting the Undersized Chin

Plastic surgeons make it a practice to avoid suggesting operations for defects of which the patient is unaware, but the one exception is the correction of a receding chin. Patients who come to the surgeon seeking a rhinoplasty (Chapter 4) may not have been conscious of the lack of balance between their nose and chin until it was pointed out to them in a profile photograph. Almost everyone is pleased with the improvement that a chin augmentation brings about. It is generally a most satisfactory operation. It is a simple procedure that in most cases has permanent results. It is done quickly, it leaves few or no conspicuous scars, and is usually free of complications. The operation may be done at the same time as the rhinoplasty and does not require additional hospitalization or convalescent time.

The procedure has been greatly simplified during recent years by the development of a number of synthetic compounds which make highly satisfactory implants, well tolerated by the body. Among them are silicone rubber and close-celled silicone sponge. The normal sensation of the chin is not affected in any way by the silicone implant.

While the search for acceptable implant material was going on, chin augmentation was accomplished mainly with cartilage or bone transplants from the patient's body. These were superior to implants of the materials then available, which gave trouble because of their unnatural consistency and their tendency to be rejected by the body. But to obtain grafts from the patient's body inflicted a second surgical wound that was often more distressing to the patient than the operation itself. Also, the bone and cartilage grafts were not completely satisfactory and frequently the chin augmentation had to be repeated once or twice over succeeding years.

In selected cases, a chin implant will correct a double chin caused by an excess of skin without any excess fat. However, the implant cannot be used to correct a chin that is too short. In order to add length to the chin, the implant would have to extend over the edge of the lower jaw and since there is no way of firmly securing the implant in this vulnerable position, it could be easily displaced. Bone grafts are more suitable for this correction because they can be wired into place.

The implant operation can be done either through the inside of the mouth, called the intraoral approach, or through a small horizontal incision underneath the chin. This is called the submental or external approach. Whether an external or internal approach is used is determined by the structure of the patient's jaw and the size of the implant needed. If the jaw is shallow or if the implant needs to be large, the surgeon may prefer the external method. The operation can be done under local anesthesia in a hospital or doctor's office and takes 30 minutes or less.

The Operation for Undersized Chin

As an added safeguard against infection and contamination, the mouth and teeth should be in as good condition as possible. Teeth should be thoroughly cleaned and scaled just prior to the operation. Some surgeons recommend brushing the teeth with an antibacterial preparation such as pHisoHex beginning a few days before surgery. Many doctors recommend antibiotics be-

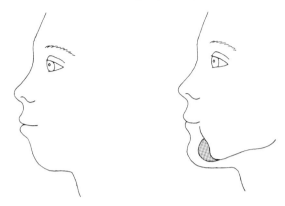

An underdeveloped chin, or microgenia, is corrected by the insertion of an implant (shaded area).

ginning two days before the operation and continuing for ten days following.

Whether the intraoral or external approach is used, the chin implant is placed in the depression between the gum and the lower lip, resting over the front surface of the mandible (lower jaw), close to the bone. There are a number of different techniques used to fashion the pocket or socket that holds the implant in place, but whatever technique is used, the ultimate aim is the same—to insert the implant in such a way that it will not be displaced and end up in the wrong position.

In one method of insertion, the surgeon makes a small incision in the depression between the gum and the lower lip. This incision is carried down to the bone and a pocket is developed, suitable in size for the implant. When the silicone rubber implant or the close-celled silicone sponge is used, it can be trimmed at the operating table to whatever size and shape are needed. The implant is then put into place and the incision is closed. Some surgeons use absorbable sutures which eventually dissolve.

Intraoral Procedure

For the submental (external) approach, an incision is made just beneath the chin in the crease that is generally present (submental crease). The incision may be less than an inch long and goes through the skin and muscle to the bone. A pocket is made close to the bone just large enough to accommodate the implant and hold it snugly in place. All bleeding points are closed off and the implant is slipped into place. Muscles and subcutaneous tissues are closed in layers and the incision is sutured. This deep closure holds the implant securely and protects the incision from splitting open.

External Approach

113

Postoperative Care

Postoperative care is the same with either the internal or external procedures. Firm dressings and adhesive tape splinting are applied to immobilize the jaw and inhibit the swelling. The dressings remain for two to four days. Once removed, they are not replaced. Antibiotics are sometimes prescribed for ten days following surgery.

Since normal chewing is hampered, the patient must have a soft or liquid diet for three days postoperatively. Analgesics may be prescribed for pain. When the external approach is used, the sutures are removed the sixth or seventh day after surgery, or at such time as the surgeon thinks appropriate.

Men should not shave for a week after the operation so as not to disturb the implant. The patient sees the doctor at weekly intervals for a few weeks, or until the doctor feels that the result is satisfactory and the patient may be discharged. Mucous membranes heal quickly and after just a few weeks, the scar inside the mouth, not being in the usual path of the tongue, is hardly discernible. The scar under the chin blends into the natural crease and in most patients is not conspicuous after several months.

Jenny S. had a chin augmentation at the same time that she had a rhinoplasty. She writes about what happened from the moment she gained consciousness and found herself back in her bed:

I'm not in <u>pain</u>, but I do feel like the man in the iron mask. A T-shaped splint is pasted tightly to my nose. A heavy chin-strap bandage is clamped tightly against the lower half of my face. My nose is packed with cotton wadding, so I can't breathe <u>that</u> way. My chin is rigid, my mouth barely open, so there's limited action <u>there</u>. I try to breathe through my ears.

I can't chew, but I can talk. The incision inside my mouth doesn't hurt, but does sting if I sip anything sharp like grapefruit juice. All diet caution to the winds, I eat ice cream and yogurt. The chin bandage will come off in three days, and the nose splint in six. A week after that, I'll be eating regular foods with only minor facial stiffness, and that will gradually disappear.

A week later . . . my new chin? It looked like a flat chunk of plaster. It was quite stiff and felt as if a wad of tunafish salad was stuck in front of my teeth and I couldn't work my tongue around to dislodge it. The implant was now "set," Dr. J. explained. The heavy bandage had flattened the chin, but, starting now, it would slowly assume a fuller, rounder shape. I couldn't wait! Both nose and chin felt tender to the touch.

Some questions came to my mind: Should I sleep on my back? . . . Was it dangerous to fly? . . . And what about sex? I could sleep any way I liked, the doctor said, though he did point out that it's <u>generally</u> better for your face—whether or not you've undergone surgery—not to sleep squashing

114

it. Flying in a commercial pressurized plane was fine unless it crashed. For another few weeks, I should try not to smash my chin during any personal entanglements. "Broom handles are the biggest danger," he added. "The most common accident occurs when you're sweeping and you hit your chin with the handle."

Everything has happened as the doctor predicted. From the front, my nose is the same length, only it's slimmer. Without the nose bump, my eyes look farther apart. The chin is rounded and natural: it adds depth to my face and, therefore, a new shape.... My profile is balanced, my nose long and straight instead of bulging out, and my chin juts out a bit instead of disappearing.... Miraculously, as the swellings have gone and the stiffness eased, I am spending less time on my looks and more time on my life. The chief effect on my new features is lightness—I feel mildly exhilarated all the time.

An extrusion, or pushing out, can occur with any solid chin implant, although perhaps not for many months or years after surgery. Careful surgery with a well-placed and well-fitted implant is the best insurance against such an occurrence. But even in the most skillfully executed operation, the implant can shift and make pressure within the mouth or on the outside of the chin. If this happens, the implant can be replaced.

However, this is not always necessary because after a period of time the chin will retain much of its new contour even without the implant. The soft tissues tend to stretch and accommodate to the presence of a foreign body and the space left by the implant tends to fill with scar tissue, so no significant change is likely to take place in the contour of the chin.

An infection would almost certainly cause an extrusion of the implant, but the use of antibiotics is a safeguard against this. There is rarely an infection in the aftermath of this operation.

If the chin implant becomes poorly positioned at any time, it can be corrected by adjusting the shape and size of the pocket.

Complications

The fee for chin augmentation ranges from $350 to $1,000. It is always performed under local anesthesia. It is purely a cosmetic procedure and is not reimbursable.

Fees

Many people think that dimples are attractive. It is pointless to speculate whether film stars Cary Grant or Kirk Douglas would have achieved their successes without the depression in the center of their chins. Undoubtedly the distinctive quality of these famous chins has made some people interested in duplicating them.

Chin dimples are generally a family characteristic, but cosmetic surgeons have tried to create them. Dimples are believed to be

Chin Dimple

115

the result of the accidental (or fortuitous, if you happen to like them) attachment of fibers from the skin to the underlying muscle. The operation to create them consists of causing an adhesion between the skin and the underlying covering of the bone (periosteum) by the careful placement of one or two sutures. The sutures remain and form a small permanent indentation by pulling the tissues inward. When a chin augmentation is performed, some surgeons advocate carving a notch in the center of the implant that will then cause an indentation in the skin of the chin that covers it. The principle behind this seems sound but many surgeons find that it is better in theory than in practice.

The results in creating artificial dimples in the cheek, using the suture method through the inside of the mouth have been quite satisfactory, but it is more difficult to copy the vertical chin furrow that a meticulous nature always places in the exact center of the chin. In spite of the surgeon's most fastidious attention to location, the handmade dimples are often not exactly centered, symmetrical, or natural in appearance and they do not move as the face moves. But even with the knowledge that the results can be less than perfect, there are patients who insist on the chin dimple and are willing to chance the consequences of a disappointing result.

Lip Reduction

Lips that are oversized or protruding can be a source of distress to many people. Most of the corrective work on deformities of the lips that plastic surgeons are called upon to perform are reconstructive procedures for conditions such as cancer of the lip or repair of harelip. But strictly within the realm of aesthetic plastic surgery, the most commonly encountered deformity is enlarged lips. They occur in varying degrees and may be congenital, a racial characteristic, or caused by inflammatory reactions, tumors, or glandular disturbances. In many cases the causes are unknown.

The surgical repair of a defect of the lips in plastic surgery is called cheiloplasty (KILE-o-plasty: *cheilos* is "lip" in Greek). In the most commonly performed method of reduction of the upper or lower lip, the surgeon removes a strip of the soft tissue that lines the inner side of the lip (mucous membrane) from one corner of the mouth to the other and sutures the wound closed. It is sometimes necessary to extend the incision well past the corners of the mouth into the lining of the cheeks. The surgery is done under local anesthesia and is a hospital procedure.

The amount of tissue removed varies in width according to the amount of reduction that is desired. There is a generous amount of tissue in the lining of the lips, so wide sections can be excised without affecting the way the lips close. This method is

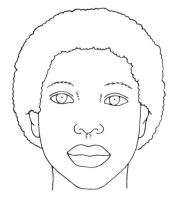

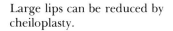

Large lips can be reduced by cheiloplasty.

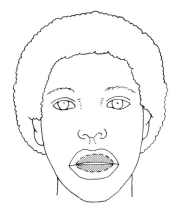

Strips of tissue are removed from the inner lining of the lips.

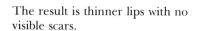

The result is thinner lips with no visible scars.

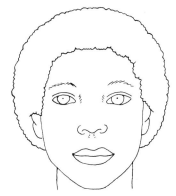

effective for reducing the lips of black people, since the incisions are in the mucous membranes and there is no danger of keloid formation.

In some patients marked swelling of the lips occurs after surgery and may persist for weeks or even months. There may be some pain for a day or two after the operation, requiring medication. A ridge of scar will remain in the mucous membrane inside the mouth, but in spite of this, patients report that the results are gratifying. Because of the initial swelling, patients may be self-conscious about returning to their usual routine for one or two weeks, even though they are quite comfortable. Patients are discharged from the hospital the day after surgery. Some surgeons use absorbable sutures and others prefer silk sutures which they may not remove until 10 or 12 days after the operation.

Another less commonly performed method of reducing a pendulous lower lip is the excision of a wedge from the center of the lip itself and the skin immediately below it. The wound is drawn together and sutured. This method leaves scars on both the lip and adjacent skin which can be concealed by lipstick and makeup. In selected cases of an enlarged lower lip, this method has been successful, but the patients must be made aware that they are exchanging a bulging lip for an improved shape and scars.

Protruding lips that are caused by protruding teeth will, of course, not be affected by a lip reduction. To achieve an improvement for this condition, the teeth would have to be repositioned either by orthodontia or surgery of the jaw, depending on the condition.

Fees   The fee for cheiloplasty ranges from $500 to $1,000.

UPPER JAWBONE
CORRECTION,
UPPER AND
LOWER TEETH
CAPPED
Before

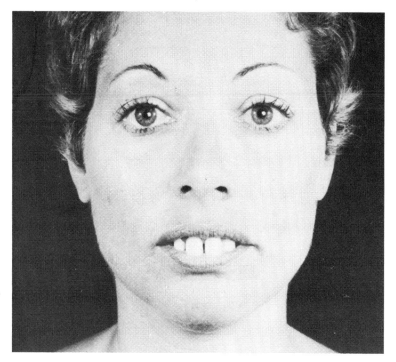

After

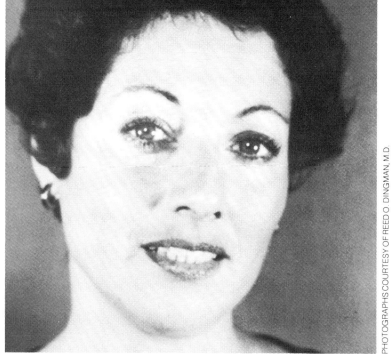

PHOTOGRAPHS COURTESY OF REED O. DINGMAN, M.D.

JAW
CORRECTION
Before

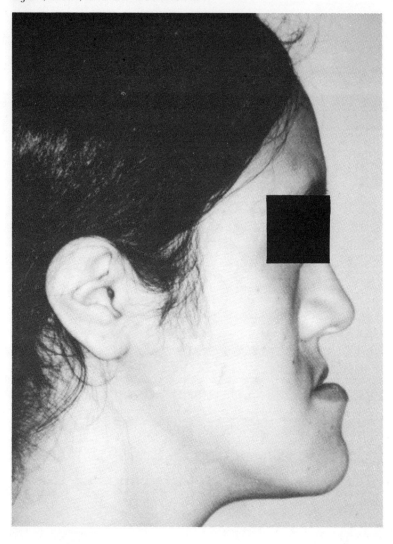

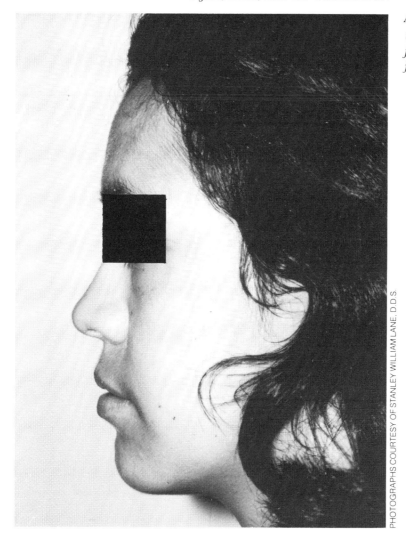

After

Upper jawbone moved forward and lower jawbone moved back.

PHOTOGRAPHS COURTESY OF STANLEY WILLIAM LANE, D.D.S.

CORRECTION OF
OPEN BITE
Before

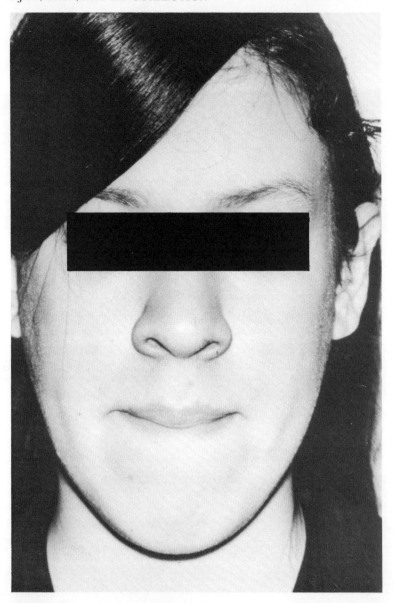

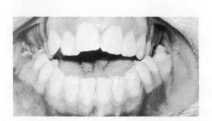

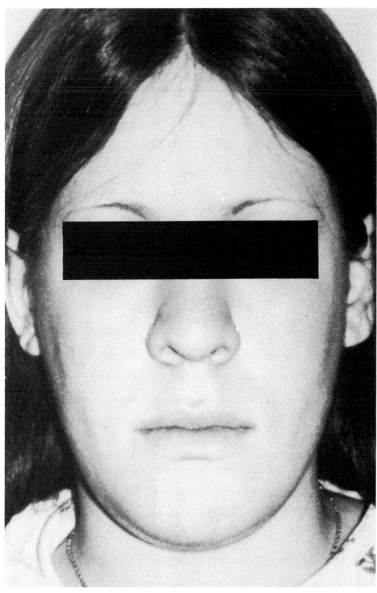

PHOTOGRAPHS COURTESY OF STANLEY WILLIAM LANE, D.D.S

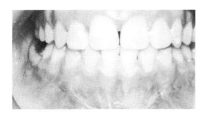

6
Ear Correction

A complex structure of hollows, planes, ridges, angles, and folds —the external ear, or auricle—is the most delicately sculpted feature on the human body. More than a mere decoration, the ear serves to capture sound waves and funnel them into the auditory canal and to protect the inner ear from damage. Acupuncturists maintain the ear also contains hundreds of tiny points that, when stimulated with needles, permit diagnosis and treatment of ailments all over the body.

The ear is a unique part of the body; no two people have ears exactly alike, nor are two ears on one person the same. Yet, despite its elegant, individual form, the ear is one of the least admired human features. Few people could accurately describe the shape of their own ears or the ears of those dear to them. Poets seldom rhapsodize over the beauties of the ear and songs are not written about it, even though the ear is the means by which poetry and song achieve their meaning.

Unfortunately, the only time the auricle gets much attention is when it is injured, missing, or deformed. Ear deformities, part of genetic inheritance, are not uncommon, and some children are born with protruding ears, lop ears, shell ears, ears buried in the head, or with one or both external ears missing. Because of its vulnerable position and fragile structure the ear is also prey to injury, sunburn, and frostbite. Older people sometimes lose an ear to cancer. Sportsmen or boxers who receive repeated blows to the ear may develop cauliflower ears—a series of hardened blood clots which make their ears bubble and swell. Some women develop keloid scarring, or cleft ear lobes, after having their ears pierced for earrings. Through injuries, parts of the ear may be severed and lost. Thus, genetic inheritance and circumstance may deform the natural configuration of the ear, making a usually anonymous feature an embarrassing focal point.

The ear is easily concealed by hair. Even men may now wear their hair over their ears and still be stylish. For people with severe ear deformities or disfigurements, however, a concealing hair style may not help a self-conscious preoccupation with a problem. For them, plastic surgeons have developed techniques for correcting various kinds of ear deformities and injuries. Some surgeons can even create a completely new ear, using cartilage and skin from other parts of the body.

Anatomy of the Ear

Development of ears begins in the human embryo in the fifth week of life as part of same tissue that eventually forms the eye and upper and lower parts of the jaw. Because the ear must undergo extensive migration during fetal development, it is susceptible to a number of hazards in the mother's womb. Intrauterine pressures or a twisted umbilical cord, for example, may damage the ear. Ear deformities are usually inherited, however, and extreme doses of the same genetic syndrome that deforms the ear may also distort the entire symmetry of the child's face.

When the child is born, the ear is fully developed and usually reaches its full size between the years of five and eight. For this reason, ears that are large on a small child may appear to shrink when the head grows to match them.

The shape and size of the human ear differs radically between individuals and between races of people. Eskimos have the longest and widest ears and blacks the shortest; in the latter, the ear lobe is small or almost absent. Caucasian ears are of medium width and are about the same length as the black ear. Japanese ear lobes are directly connected to the skin of the upper neck.

The elaborate planes and configurations of the ear provide a buttress that holds the shell-like structure in the proper relationship to the head. The normal ear is situated between the eyebrows and the base of the nose and is attached to the head at an angle of 30 degrees. If the angle is wider, the ear protrudes; the greater the angle, the greater the degree of protrusion. The ear is composed of a tough elastic cartilage, encased in a fibrous cover called the perichondrium, which in turn is covered with a thin, adherent layer of skin. Because almost no fat lies between the skin of the ear and the cartilage, the ear is easily affected by temperature changes. Only the lobe of the ear, reputedly an erogenous zone, contains subcutaneous tissue and no cartilage. The skin behind the ear, which matches the skin of the face closely in color and texture, is used for skin grafts. Weak vestigial muscles are located on the outside of the auricle and can still be used by some people to wiggle the ears.

Each angle, protrusion, and concavity of the ear has a medical designation. The helix is a tubular rim which runs from the top of the ear to the edge of the lobe; the antihelix is the gracefully curved tube of cartilage which gives the ear its shape; the scapha is the furrow separating the helix and the antihelix; the concha is

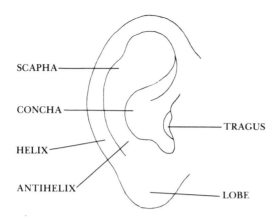

SCAPHA

CONCHA

HELIX

ANTIHELIX

TRAGUS

LOBE

ANATOMY OF THE EAR

the shell-shaped concavity of the ear leading to the auditory canal; and the tragus is the small protrusion on the outside of the concha close to the face.

There are many different kinds of ear deformities and no two deformities, like no two ears, are exactly alike. Sometimes the deformity afflicts one ear and not the other, or in some cases the ears may be deformed differently on each side of the head. Some people suffer from a combination of deformities.

Ear Deformities

The most common ear deformity is a "protruding ear," or an ear which springs out from the scalp instead of lying a short distance away. Most ears protrude because of faulty development of the antihelix—the fold of cartilage that gives the ear its characteristic shape and bends it toward the head. When this fold is poorly formed or absent, causing the cartilage of the ear

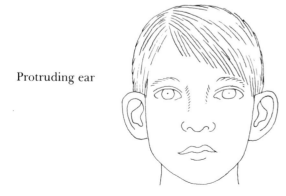

Protruding ear

127

to lie flat instead of in a furled position, the "spring" which pulls the ear toward the head is missing and the ear sticks out. Parents used to try to correct a child's protruding ears by sticking them to the head with adhesive tape or pinning them back with caps of various kinds. The dauntless elastic ear cartilage, however, will not be restrained by nonsurgical methods.

Protruding ears often appear too large because of their prominent position framing the face, but once they are restructured and placed in a more natural position they are revealed to be of a normal size. Some ears protrude, however, because there is an excess of cartilage in the concha, or because there is a disparity in size between the rim of the helix and the conchal rim. These ears are called "cupped ears," or "telephone ears," because the ear appears as if it were being cupped to receive incoming sounds.

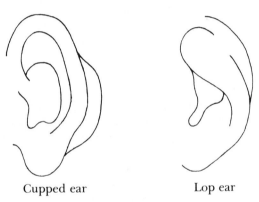

Cupped ear   Lop ear

Because of the shape of the ear, the height from the top to the lobe may appear reduced. A "lop ear," another type of deformity, is so called because the top of the helix and scapha fold downward. A lop ear may also protrude and appear too small. Sometimes lopped and cupped ears *are* too small—modified forms of an ear deformity called microtia, or missing ear. In its severest form, microtia is a congenital defect in which there is only a knot of skin and cartilage instead of a normal ear.

Other ear deformities, though comparatively rare, include "shell ears," or flat ears without the helix rim; "invaginated ears," or ears partially embedded in the scalp; and "satyr ears," or ears with a devilish point to the helix. The ear may also be too large or have too long a lobe.

All ear deformities are inherited, and the gene which causes them may be either dominant or recessive. If both parents suffer from ear deformities, the chances are great that their children will be born with one or more deformities which may be more severe than in either of the parents.

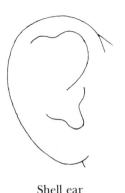

Shell ear

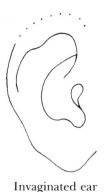

Invaginated ear

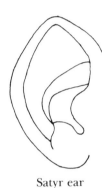

Satyr ear

Ear deformities are associated with no medical problems, although sometimes people born without an ear suffer hearing loss. The deformity may, nevertheless, become a source of misery to the afflicted person. Many years ago in Europe, innocent people were arrested because police were taught that abnormalities of the external ear indicated the criminally insane. Children with protruding ears are frequently taunted by their playmates, and nicknames such as "Dumbo," "Bat Ears," "Donkey Ears," and "Mickey Mouse" are not unknown to them.

Surgery to correct deformed ears, or otoplasty, has been performed since the 19th Century. The first American operation to correct the most common deformity, the protruding ear, was performed in New York in 1881. The first otoplasties were done by removing a wedge of skin from the back of the ear, then suturing the ear to the head to hold it there. The procedure was ineffective because the tough, elastic ear cartilage resisted the sutures and soon propelled the ears back to their former position. Moreover, ears sutured to the head look as bizarre in their plastered-back position as do protruding ears.

Surgery for Protruding Ears

129

In this century, plastic surgeons have successfully developed countless techniques for correcting the protruding ear. One surgeon estimates that medical literature describes nearly 200 techniques for the operation, some differing only slightly from one another. Each surgeon has his own method and may vary the operation according to the ear he is working on. A protruding ear that is also cupped or lopped requires different techniques than an ear that protrudes simply because the antihelix is not well developed. Doctors use the technique they feel most comfortable with and the one that gives the best results. One surgeon said:

I'm not so gung ho on my technique, but since it gives me good results I don't see any reason to change it. A surgeon can correct protruding ears by a number of methods. The important thing is the result, not the method.

All the procedures used to correct the protruding ear, though technically different, evolve from the same principle: a protruding ear suffers from an abnormal configuration of ear cartilage and that cartilage must be weakened, removed, or stitched into a more aesthetic position to create a properly positioned ear.

The Consultation   The primary reason to operate on a deformed ear is to eliminate the psychological trauma the defect may cause. Children usually suffer the most from protruding ears, because other children tease them about their deformity. Adults often seek ear correction also. Men and women whose ears were not corrected as children may still bear the lingering effect of childhood trauma and remain self-conscious about their disfigurations.

Hair styles are limited in people embarrassed by ear deformities, and severely protruding ears may emerge from behind even the longest concealing locks. Men, who usually prefer short styles, may be especially self-conscious about the problem. Lately, however, it has become fashionable for young boys, the worst victims of traumatizing insults, to wear their hair longer and disguise defective ears. According to one surgeon, the number of parents requesting ear correction for small boys is on the wane for this reason. Sometimes, however, women with protruding ears feel unable to wear their hair in becoming short styles or upswept hairdos. Said one otoplastic patient, Hannah, age 34:

I can't remember other children teasing me about my protruding ears when I was small, probably because my mother would never let me wear my hair in braids or a ponytail. She had a complex about her own

130

protruding ears and passed it on to me. I got the distinct impression from her that something was wrong with my ears, and after a while I became extremely self-conscious about them.

I've spent countless hours in the last 20 years designing long, curly, bouffant styles that would keep my ears hidden. All the time what I really wanted was a short cut. I'm a nurse in a hospital and I met a patient who had had her ears corrected. I contacted the same surgeon and had mine done right away. Maybe nobody notices my new ears, but I'm happy I no longer have to notice them either. I now have a gorgeous, short French cut from one of the best salons. It is easy to care for and needs no curlers.

Adults tormented about protruding ears as children, like Hannah's mother, may project their own feelings to their sons or daughters. Since ear defects are hereditary, the parent who brings his child to the surgeon may bear the same protruding ears. One doctor said:

I've had situations where a father with protruding ears doesn't want his child to go through the same torment. When I talk to the child, however, it's apparent he is not at all tormented. If the child does not seem to care if his or her ears protrude, I don't do the operation.

Another surgeon stated:

If other children are making fun of a child with protruding ears and he's aware of it, I do the operation. If the ears don't bother the child, I don't do it. Whether or not to do the ears should be the child's decision. I talk to the child as I would to any patient to determine his motivation.

Adults seeking otoplasty should also be motivated and should realize that otoplasty, like all plastic procedures, will not change their lives fundamentally.

No aspirin or aspirin-containing medicine should be taken two weeks before the operation. Most ear operations are performed in a hospital. Local anesthesia is usually sufficient for patients over ten. If the patient is a young child or apprehensive about the operation, general anesthesia is recommended.

Preoperative Procedures

The doctor first examines the patient's ears and determines the best method to correct them by carefully evaluating the anatomical reasons for the protrusion. The operative area is thoroughly cleansed and draped and the ears exposed through openings in a sterile stockinette. If the patient has long hair, it is fastened back and above the ears. The hair is never cut or shaved.

The incision to expose the ear cartilage is usually made on the

131

back of the ear to eliminate the possibility of scars. Some doctors make the incision on the front of the ear in the concealing demarcation between the helix and the antihelix. In both instances, the doctor bends the ear back to produce a fold, then outlines the incision he plans to make with dye.

Surgical
Procedure

All surgical procedures for correcting protruding ears attempt to remold or to eliminate excess or defectively formed cartilage that causes the ear to protrude. Since the architectural construction and stress of the elastic fibers on the front and back of the cartilage create the shape of the ear, it is these fibers that must be weakened or reshaped to correct the ear's position. The surgeon may:

1. Divide or weaken the fibers on the front of the cartilage so the natural pull of the fibers on the back will have more power to bend the ear toward the head. In general, when the surgeon cuts or weakens ear cartilage on one side, the ear will bend toward the side where the cartilage remains intact. To weaken the cartilage, the surgeon severs, scores, or thins it with an instrument similar to a fine razor blade or with an electrically rotating wire brush. Basically, he is attempting to break the spring of the cartilage which propels the ear forward.

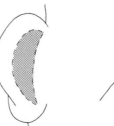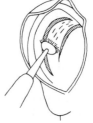

For correction of protruding ears, skin on the back of the ear is excised (shaded area). The back of the ear is abraded to make the cartilage thinner and more flexible.

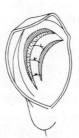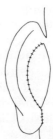

The cartilage is rolled and sutured to form the antihelix. The final sutures are made.

2. Once the spring of the cartilage is broken, the surgeon may suture it into the shape of a tube, or antihelix. The nonabsorbable sutures are buried in the cartilage and hold the ear permanently in the desired shape. Children whose ear cartilage is tender and malleable may not need to have the spring broken before the cartilage is tubed. The cartilage in adult ears is tougher, and more effort is used to break it down before molding it into the desired shape. Sometimes it is sufficient just to break the spring of the cartilage without creating an artificial antihelical fold with sutures.

3. If there is excess cartilage, the surgeon may remove part of it.

In order to reveal the cartilage, the surgeon undermines the skin, or lifts it from the surface of the cartilage, on whatever side of the ear he is working on. After the operation the incision line is sutured.

If the top and bottom of the ear still protrude after the cartilage in the body of the ear is corrected, additional procedures are needed to bring the ear into balance. The surgeon may continue the incision further down the ear toward the lobe, or remove excess tissue in the lobe. If the top of the ear still projects forward, a small piece of horizontal helix is excised.

Once one of the patient's ears is corrected, the other one will often seem to protrude. Therefore, most surgeons plan to operate on both ears in the same procedure.

Postoperative Procedures

Otoplasty patients remain in the hospital for one day. Various types of turban dressings are used and the concavities of the ear are packed with moist padding. This dressing is changed after one day and is worn for four to seven days after the operation. Sometimes doctors recommend that an elastic headband be worn at night to maintain the position of the ears during sleep for one or two weeks. Since the operation itself permanently corrects protruding ears, dressings are not what hold them in place.

Otoplasty patients should not expose ears to the sun or temperature extremes for one month after the operation. Hair can be washed after a week. The ears remain a violet color for approximately one month, and slight swelling for several weeks is normal. Activities that might cause injury to the ear should be avoided.

Possible Complications

The most common complication of otoplasty is accumulation of blood in the ear, or clotting; the blood must be evacuated by the doctor. Persistent pain under the dressing is a warning. Since infection is a possible side effect of clotting, large doses of antibiotics are often given when this condition occurs. Infection, however, is extremely uncommon. Hypertrophic scarring and keloid scars may occur in some people.

A poor cosmetic result is the most frequent complication of otoplasty. The ear should be set at a proper distance from the head, not too close and not too far away. Ridges, irregularities, or sharp edges should not appear on the ear surface, and the lobe and top of the ear should be in the correct position. Patients should not expect both of their ears to look exactly the same after surgery because ears are never the same to begin with. The profile, too, only shows one ear at a time, so no one notices ears that don't match. In general, surgeons are much more aware of the less-than-perfect results of otoplasty than their patients who can't see their ears very well anyway. As long as the ear no longer protrudes and looks natural, the patient is usually satisfied.

Fees

Fees for the various kinds of otoplasty range from $750 to $1,500, depending on the amount of correction and the part of the country where the operation is performed.

Correction of Other Ear Deformities

Lop ear. When the helix and scapha droop or hang downward, the helix is too short to allow the ear to be raised into a normal position. The surgeon has techniques to lengthen the tissue of the helix and raise the ear. The cartilage of the drooping fold may be weakened to help keep the ear upright.

Cup ear. Cupped ears usually protrude and may have excess cartilage in the concha, which is removed. Cupped ears may also be sutured to the head.

Shell ear. Shell ears lack the helix, or rim of the ear, almost entirely. Surgeons correct the deformity by thinning the cartilage along the back edge of the ear, which causes the tissue to curl forward. The edge of the ear may then be rolled and sutured in the shape of a helix.

Satyr ear. The point in the helix of satyr ears is caused by incomplete curling at some place along the helix rim. The pointed section can be trimmed, or tubed and sutured into shape.

Invaginated ear. Ears attached to the scalp or half buried in it prevent the wearing of glasses. To correct this deformity, the surgeon releases the upper part of the ear from the scalp and applies skin grafts to the denuded back of the ear.

Macrotia. As long as the ear is set at an angle close to the scalp it seldom appears oversized. In cases where ears are exceptionally large (macrotia), surgeons excise wedges of tissue in varying shapes and close the empty space with sutures. There are, however, few requests to reduce ear size in nonprotruding ears. The same kind of cut-and-suture technique can also alter the size of the lobes.

Microtia. Once in every 20,000 births a child is born without one or both external ears. Microtia, as it is called, also designates a reduced and deformed ear mass. Hearing damage may occur in severe cases. The ear may be replaced by surgical methods or with a prosthetic ear.

Ear Replacement

For people born without an ear or for those who have lost an ear as a result of accident or disease, plastic surgeons have developed a highly complex series of procedures through which an artificial ear is created from skin and cartilage grafts from the patient's own body. Although many surgeons have tried ear replacement procedures with some success, few are experts. The resulting ear, depending on the surgeon's skill, is better than no ear at all, but may not exactly resemble a natural auricle. In general, the reconstructed ear is heavier and bulkier than the natural ear and lacks its sculpted configurations. As one doctor put it, "It's hard to create something from nothing."

To reconstruct an ear, the surgeon first does a reverse tracing of the opposite ear (if it exists) in order to have a model for the new one. In the first procedure, cartilage is excised from another part of the patient's body, usually the rib cage, and carved in the shape of a basic ear structure by the surgeon. Then this ear framework is placed in a vertical incision or pocket which has been created in the patient's head to hold it. Some surgeons prefer to use a silicone implant instead of rib cartilage to create the basic framework for the new ear. The patient's body, however, may not tolerate the artificial substance. The skin is encouraged to adhere to the ear framework with the help of sutures. The ear lobe, usually present in microtia, is rotated and sutured into a horizontal position in a procedure done before or at the same time that the ear framework is implanted.

Weeks later, when the skin seems to be adhering to the framework, the ear is resurrected from the pocket and skin is grafted onto raw surfaces. About four months are needed for these grafts to adhere. Later, in subsequent procedures, the surgeon creates approximations of the other planes and elevations of the ear with additional skin grafts. Fees for a surgical ear replacement are about $2,000. If more than one ear is reconstructed, a rare occurrence, the fee is about $3,000.

Prosthetic Ears

Prosthetic ears, created from new plastic materials, such as silicone rubbers and polyvinyl chloride, are now extremely sophisticated, thanks to new techniques for molding and coloring plastics. People who have lost an ear through injury or disease, or who were born without an ear, often prefer a prosthetic ear to a surgically reconstructed one. Although the prosthetic ear is not a living part of the person as the reconstructed ear is, it usually bears a greater resemblance to the natural human auricle. Surgery may not be desirable for people who are old or in poor health, or who have lost an ear as a result of malignancy. Often there may be no plastic surgeon available who is trained in the reconstruction operation.

Initially the patient is recommended to a prosthetist by his doctor. The prosthetist examines the site of the missing ear and makes an impression of both sides of the head. If there is redundant tissue from unsuccessful reconstructive surgery or if part of an ear is present, it may have to be removed surgically before the prosthesis can be fitted to the head. Since only one ear is usually missing, the prosthetist models the new ear on the existing ear. First he makes a rough sculpture of the new auricle, then tests its alignment and appearance on the patient's head. Later, the ear is sculpted more finely and colored to match the patient's skin by an artist with an airbrush. Fine details and skin markings are added. Then a final mold of the new ear, which can be used to create replacements, is cast.

The prosthetic ear may be attached by a number of methods. Usually a liquid adhesive is used, but the ear may also be attached surgically by means of pockets created in the head, and skin bridges. When the ear is attached with adhesive, it should be removed at least every few days so the area beneath it can be washed. The prosthetic ear may also be attached to the frames of glasses. The prosthetic ear is not always practical for children or extremely active adults as it may fall off at embarrassing moments.

Tailor-made prosthetic ears are now very expensive—often more than $2,000 for the creation of the permanent mold and first prosthesis. But once the mold is established, replacements are inexpensive. Replacements are needed when the tissue beneath the prosthesis changes size. If the original ear is missing completely, few replacements are needed in the patient's lifetime. State institutes of vocational rehabilitation often pay for prosthetic devices.

Correction of Ear Injuries

Cauliflower ear. Cauliflower ears occur from blows to the ear and are often found on boxers. The ear begins bleeding on the inside and the blood clots. If the blood is not evacuated immediately by a surgeon, it can become hard and fibrous and eventually harden the cartilage. Ideally, the surgeon evacuates the blood before it organizes and inflames the cartilage; but once the lumps that give the deformity the name of cauliflower have permanently formed, the surgeon must shave the cartilage in order to thin it out. The deformity is hard to treat and makes the ear look small and disfigured.

Cut or severed ear. Sometimes part of the ear is severed in an accident. If the piece is rescued and available to the surgeon, he can graft it to the back of the ear to reestablish its blood supply. Later he can replant it in its proper position. Other grafts can be substituted for the missing piece.

Injuries resulting from pierced ears. Although thousands of people have their ears pierced for earrings without any problems, injuries or scars develop in a significant number. The lobe of the ear may become cleft if the ear is pierced too low or if the earring is pulled or passes through the lobe. The surgeon must excise part of the lobe and restitch it to correct the cleft. Cysts, too, may develop after ear piercing, and people with keloid tendencies may form huge scar growths after the ears are pierced. Keloids may also form after ear surgery. Although treating keloids is difficult, a measure of success is sometimes obtained by injecting the keloid formation with steroids. Radiation, too, is sometimes effective if it is done immediately after scar correction.

Finding a Surgeon for Otoplasty

Otoplasty is always done by a plastic surgeon. Sometimes a plastic surgeon and an otolaryngologist work together when hearing problems exist with cosmetic deformities. The majority of plastic surgeons are familiar with correction procedures for protruding ears and other minor deformities, but there may be fewer surgeons familiar with more complicated procedures, such as reconstruction of a missing ear. Most reputable surgeons will refer patients to an experienced doctor if they don't know how to do the requested otoplasty. Generally, a university medical school hospital has doctors on the staff who have corrected all kinds of ear deformities.

**CORRECTION OF
DEFORMED AND
PROTRUDING
EARS**

Before

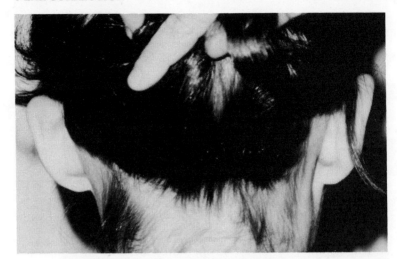

After

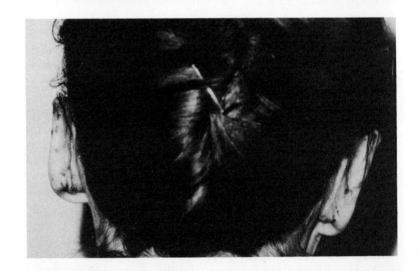

Side view

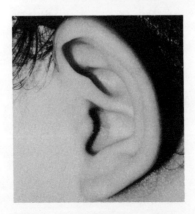 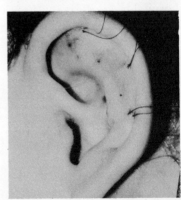

PHOTOGRAPHS COURTESY OF PETER LINDEN, M.D.

7

Skin Improvement:

Removal of wrinkles, lines, moles, scars, and other imperfections

From childhood on, our skins serve as a living record of the passage of time. No one fully understands the biochemical process that leads to aging of the skin, but no one past 35 fails to understand the initial signs of the process—those first faint lines that etch the face with the promise of things to come. What happens over the years to the silky soft, smooth, poreless skin in which we were originally packaged depends on many factors. Some are beyond our control, others are not. No matter what we do, the skin will inevitably lose some of its elasticity and velvety texture. It will wrinkle and sag, and patches of pigmentation may appear, but there are measures that may be taken to help delay these changes.

Time alone, however, is not always responsible for the premature signs of aging. They can be connected with a variety of other causes ranging from a family characteristic to debilitating disease and mental and physical stress. The greatest offender in the aging and deterioration of the skin in most Caucasians is self-inflicted—through excessive exposure to the sun. It is as basic and simple as that. Many of the skin problems brought to the plastic surgeon are the direct result of this overindulgence.

Overexposure to the Sun

There is nothing new about sun worship. It has been going on since prehistoric times. In various cultures the sun was deified and placated with human sacrifices. Judging from some of the thickened, leathery faces now seen about, one might suspect that this practice is continuing.

How would you explain why people who draw the shades and tilt the blinds in their houses so their furniture, curtains, and carpets won't dry out, crack, or fade (and thus look good a bit longer) could ignore taking the same precautions with their own precious and irreplaceable skin? Indifferent to the warnings of the irreversible skin damage that the cumulative effects of the sun can cause in later life, they vigorously pursue the sun winter

140

and summer with ever-dwindling areas of their bodies under cover. People in the desert who swathe themselves in voluminous burnooses for protection against the sun exhibit considerably better judgment than the hordes of scantily clad sun worshipers in our Western world who roast their skins for the sake of a tan.

Although the glow of a suntanned skin may present an image of vigor and vitality, the adverse effects of acquiring that tan too often outweigh the advantages. Tanning does not signify health; it is merely the reaction of the skin seeking to protect itself from the rays of the sun. The only beneficial effects of tanning, aside from the psychological feeling of well-being, is the formation of vitamin D, which is adequately provided in the normal American diet. On the other hand, continued exposure to the sun's rays can result in the breakdown of tissues, cellular damage, irregular pigmentation, and irreversible degenerative changes in the skin, leading to precancerous and cancerous skin conditions. It might be noted that about 90 percent of skin cancers are on exposed areas, especially the face. Skin cancer is rare in black people who are also less susceptible to sunburn. Statistics indicate that in the United States there is more skin cancer in the southern states, where there is also more sunshine than in other sections of the country.

The effects of sun on skin are not conjectural. Laboratory studies of human skin samples have demonstrated the effects of repeated assaults of sun. Skin from the face of older persons was compared with skin from other parts of the body not normally exposed. The body skin preserved much of the fiber quality of healthy young tissue while the facial skin in the same persons showed marked deterioration. Collagen is the main supportive protein found in the skin, tendon, bone, cartilage, and connective tissue. In the exposed sun-damaged skin the total collagen content was decreased and altered, making the skin appear older than its chronological age.

Skin varies greatly in the amount of sun it can tolerate. You must determine for yourself how much sun you can be exposed to comfortably. Melanin is the dark pigment in the skin that is chiefly responsible for its color. The darker the skin, the more melanin it contains and the longer it can resist the sun's rays without becoming inflamed. Dark-skinned, dark-haired, dark-eyed people generally have greater tolerance to sunlight than blond or red-haired people with blue eyes and fair skins. Black skin has many times the Caucasian's protection against permanent damage and skin cancer. The response to the sun's rays can vary from a slight redness to severe burn with swelling, blistering, and a general feeling of illness. Some skins react by freckling. Freckles may appear after initial exposure to the sun and remain for several months or permanently. Freckles do not appear in skin that has not been exposed to sunlight.

Sense in the Sun

Protecting your skin against the effects of overexposure to the sun does not mean that you must forever hide in a tent. No one who goes outdoors in the summer can possibly avoid the sun's rays. They are reflected back at you from sidewalks and buildings. But there are simple precautions you can take to minimize overexposure. An effective program would include a combination of proper clothing, protective face makeup, and moderation in the time spent in the direct sunlight. Bear in mind that the intensity of the sun varies. It is greater in summer than in winter. It is more powerful at high altitudes than at sea level and in tropical climates than in temperate zones; it is at its peak between 11 a.m. and 3 p.m. Not even a milky-skinned blond is likely to get a sunburn before 8 o'clock in the morning or after 4 o'clock in the afternoon.

City or country dwellers who are going to be in the midday sun for any length of time would do well to wear a broad-brimmed hat and long sleeves. The large-brimmed hats worn by North American cowboys and South American gauchos did not spring from a designer's caprice, but out of need for protection from the sun.

Sunscreen Preparations

A wide variety of protective skin products known as sun blocks and sunscreens afford differing degrees of protection from ultraviolet radiation. In spite of some extravagant claims made by their manufacturers, they must be selected with care according to the needs of your skin and with an eye on the list of ingredients.

The greatest amount of protection is given by preparations containing opaque chemicals such as zinc oxide or titanium dioxide, which actually create a barrier between your skin and the sun's ultraviolet rays. They are known as sun blocks. They are effective, but are mostly for limited supersentitive areas such as the nose, cheeks, and forehead and are not aesthetically pleasing.

A high degree of protection is afforded by suntan lotions or creams containing chemicals known as sunscreeens, which absorb wavelengths of the burning ultraviolet rays of sunlight. The most effective chemicals in these sunscreens are either PABA (para-aminobenzoic acid) or sulisobenzone. Many of the popular sunscreen preparations use one or the other and each is highly desirable. The more valuable preparations allow you to stay in the sun longer with less risk of burning, but none is 100 percent

142

effective. Do not allow yourself to be lulled into a false sense of security after one application. Suntan products must be reapplied every few hours, after each swim, and whenever the protective film may have rubbed off or washed away.

Makeup preparations containing sunscreens are limited in the protection they offer unless they are opaque or contain 5 percent PABA, in which case they are excellent. But even makeup products with minimal sunscreens are better than no protection at all and can be recommended for that reason. In any case no one should depend on any sunscreen preparation to provide complete protection from intensive sunlight or for all-day exposure.

The lips may also react to too much sun. Again, prevention is the important consideration. Lipstick provides significant protection for women. Topical sunscreens in the form of colorless lipstick can be used by either men or women.

After sunbathing and before going to bed always use an emollient lotion or cream on your skin. It will not prevent or reverse the damage from overexposure to the sun but it will counteract the drying effect of the sun.

A Safe Glow

It is scarcely necessary to talk about the foolhardiness of roasting all day in the sun for a single weekend in order to end up with a tan. If you have only a weekend to spare for this project, you will do well to forget about a tan and buy a skin bronzer or darker makeup.

Suntans must be acquired slowly and gradually. People with fair skin should limit their first exposure to no more than 15 to 20 minutes of sun for each side of the body, and even less in the tropics. Exposure time can be increased by about one-third each day. After a week there should be enough new pigment in the skin to protect it against burning.

Do not depend on a beach umbrella for safety from the sun. Rays reflected from sand and water can burn even when you are indirectly exposed. Hazy, foggy or overcast days must also be suspect because these atmospheric conditions scatter the sun's burning rays and may produce severe sunburn.

The same precautions must be observed on a skiing vacation, which can be as searing as an interlude on a sun-baked tropical island. Not only is the sun stronger at higher altitudes, but additional radiation is reflected by the snow, increasing the hazard of sunburn.

Skin Care

Even if all of the extravagant claims made by the cosmetic industry touting facial lotions, oils, drops, and creams that erase the tracks of time cannot be substantiated, they should not be completely dismissed. The purpose of these products, called moisturizers, lubricators, night creams, and so on, is to prevent or counteract signs and symptoms of skin dryness. They are all emollients—products that soften and soothe the skin. When skin is dry, it becomes chapped and rough. It is the loss of water, not oil, from the outer layer of the skin that is the basic cause of dryness. Moisture content is essential to maintaining a youthful skin, although it should be understood that dryness is not the cause of permanent wrinkles.

Most of the preparations are mixtures of oil and water with other ingredients added to prevent spoilage, to keep the oil and water in suspension, and to provide a scent. Some of the water in these lotions or creams evaporates when applied, but the oily film left on the skin retards the evaporation of moisture from the outer layer of the skin and helps to keep the skin soft and flexible. They also improve the appearance of the skin by soothing the rough, scaly surface.

There is a wide selection of such products from which to choose. Many different kinds of oil, some with exotic histories and origins—mink, turtle, placenta extract, and royal jelly, among others— are used, but there is no evidence that one kind is better than another. Select whatever product pleases you in terms of its consistency, fragrance, and cost, and use it faithfully. They will all be of some help. Even women who live in a moist, humid climate are well advised to use a moisturizer as they go into their fourth decade. The 16-year-old can get by with a freshly scrubbed face and a dash of lip gloss, but the older skin needs a lot more help and attention.

All of these emollient creams are variations on the formula for old-fashioned cold cream, but they have been modified so that their primary purpose is to smooth and soften rather than to cleanse. Since they are meant to remain on the skin instead of being wiped off like cold cream, they are made less greasy. Cold cream has been around since the 2nd Century when the great Greek physician Galen is believed by some historians to have invented it. The original formula consisted of olive oil, beeswax, and water, with some rose petals added for fragrance. It was called cold cream because when it was applied to the skin the water evaporated, producing a cool feeling. Many women still prefer cold cream to other creams, and use it both for cleansing and lubricating.

Wrinkles, Lines, Scars, and Other Imperfections

Even when we have taken the most exquisite care of our skin—not baking it or broiling it, not abusing it or neglecting it—and have gone so far as to choose ancestors who aged well, the time must come for all of us when wrinkles and wattles, pouches, and

144

pigmentations make their unwelcome appearance. Aesthetic surgery offers a trio of procedures for dealing with these conditions. They may not restore an unblemished, unlined skin, but they have been highly effective in improving it. The procedures are the face lift, which redrapes the skin; dermabrasion or chemical peeling, which resurfaces it; and injections of liquid silicone, which adds tissue volume, filling out wrinkles not affected by the first two procedures.

Dermabrasion, a mechanical scraping of the skin surface, has been effective in lessening light wrinkles and in improving the appearance of scars and pits that remain after severe acne. It will not remove the scars but, by abrading the high points or elevations so that the low ones appear less deep, it makes them less noticeable. Chemical peeling has been successful in the treatment of certain types of wrinkles and facial pigmentations. It achieves its purpose by the use of a solution of chemicals that, in effect, burns away the top layers of the skin. The method of choice is determined by the surgeon or dermatologist and the condition of the skin.

Only physicians trained in the technique of these procedures should perform them. They should never be done by a lay person or in a commercial "beauty clinic" that advertises. The operations are not simple, quick, or painless. They require skill and extensive training. In improper hands, unsightly scarring and permanent damage can result. The choice of patients for these operations is also important, for not every patient who is interested is suitable, and judicious selection of patients, which can be done only by an experienced physician, is essential.

Skin planing, or dermabrasion, is a technique for the removal of the outer layers of the skin with a rapidly rotating wire brush or burr. It results in a smoothing of the surface irregularities of the skin. Dermabrasion evolved primarily to improve skins scarred and pitted by acne, but it can also be useful in alleviating fine lines and shallow wrinkles, removing freckles and other skin pigmentations, and treating premalignant lesions in skin damaged by overexposure to sun.

Dermabrasion

The degree of improvement achieved depends upon the pathology being dealt with. A skin with deep diffuse scars does not respond as well as one with shallow craters and well-defined pits. In many cases, the results can be most gratifying and even dramatic, but patients are cautioned not to expect their skin to be restored to its pristine smoothness, free of defects. They may rightfully look forward to improvement but not a miracle, and should view the results in relation to the previous condition.

Generally, one planing is sufficient for fine lines, wrinkles, freckles, and superficial pigmentations. But scarring from acne, chicken pox, or smallpox may need two or three procedures. Only a superficial or intermediate thickness of skin surface can be abraded at one time, for if the skin planing is too deep, it can itself generate scars and increase the always-present danger of irregular pigmentation. The skin regenerates almost entirely, however, and the procedure may be repeated after a rest period of from three to six months, depending on the patient's healing ability. The first dermabrasion results in a greater improvement, proportionately, than the repeated dermabrasions.

There are certain conditions and kinds of skins that are unlikely prospects for successful planing. Large-pored skin is not improved. Pores are too deep to be reached without damaging healthy tissue, and a superficial planing does not affect them. Dermabrasion is not recommended in the regions of the neck, chest, back, legs, and feet because skin regeneration is slow in these parts of the body. Besides the delay in healing, there is danger of excessive scarring. Any skin with a tendency to keloid formation (heavy scars) is also out of bounds for dermabrasion for obvious reasons. People with dark skins are poor risks not only because of the danger of keloid formation but also because of the possibility of a marked change in pigmentation after planing.

There is no age limit for patients whose skins could be benefited by dermabrasion. Teenagers and people in their sixties may be treated, although the older person may take a little longer to heal. In the opinion of some specialists, dermabrasion may be performed on young people during the active stages of acne with beneficial results.

How the Technique of Skin Planing Evolved

In ancient times, beauty-conscious Egyptian women used an abrasive paste made of particles of alabaster mixed with honey and milk to smooth their skins. Now, 3,500 years later, abrasive creams and synthetic and genuine sponges with rough surfaces are still being used for the same purpose.

Mechanical abrasion of the skin for the removal of superficial lesions was first introduced in the 1900s. Initially it was done with cylindrical knives, which were later replaced by mechanically driven dental burrs and rasps, a kind of coarse file. The skin was sometimes—not always—anesthetized.

In 1935 the use of a wire brush to abrade the skin was reported and interest in the technique gradually developed. The traumatic tattoos from gunpowder suffered by many soldiers during World War II heightened the need for extensive abrasive therapy. Sandpaper came into use in treating these foreign-body tattoo injuries and later it was borrowed for the removal of freckles and scars. But this was only the beginning. Since the 1950s, instruments have been developed that have greatly refined the techniques of mechanical skin planing. In one of the most widely used methods, a motor-driven instrument revolves at a high speed (24,000 revolutions per minute) and is controlled by varying the pressure on a foot pedal. To it is attached a wire brush or diamond-impregnated burr with which the surface layers of the skin are scraped away.

The Operation

Some physicians perform dermabrasion in the office using local anesthesia. Others prefer general anesthesia in a hospital. As would be expected, each school has valid reasons for its choice. The actual procedure and postoperative course are the same in either situation and, as we know, there can be many pathways to a good result. Patients must have confidence that their surgeon is using a technique that has worked well for him and for his other patients. Hospitalized patients are discharged the day following the operation.

Preparation

As in all cosmetic surgery, before-and-after photographs may be required. Aspirin or products containing aspirin should not be taken for two weeks before the operation because the drug tends to promote bleeding. The hair should be shampooed the evening before. Men are asked to shave as closely as possible on the day of the operation.

When abrasion is performed in the doctor's office, women patients are asked to wear comfortable clothing that need not be pulled over the head after the operation so that dressings or the operated area are not disturbed. Patients should always have someone with them to accompany them home afterwards.

Surgical Procedure

When the operation is done under local anesthesia, the patients are premedicated so they will be thoroughly relaxed. The face is carefully cleansed and, depending on the surgeon's choice, either injected with a local anesthetic or sprayed with a topical spray, such as ethyl chloride or Freon, which has a freezing action. This spray anesthetizes the skin, firms it, and minimizes the bleeding. Its anesthetic action is very short—15 to 30 seconds—so the face is anesthetized and abraded in small sections. After one area is treated, another is anesthetized and abraded. The procedure is repeated until the entire face is done. The abrading is usually carried well into the temple and hairline region and just beneath the jawline so there will be no contrast in color between the planed and unplaned areas. A full face abrasion may take from 20 to 40 minutes, depending on how fast the physician works.

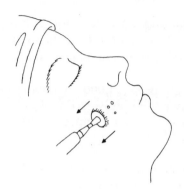

Dermabrasion removes the outer layers of the skin with a wire brush revolving at tremendously high speed.

There is some pain or discomfort while the skin is being frozen and when it thaws, but there is no pain during the abrading process itself. Immediately after the operation, an anesthetic solution is applied to the face to reduce the burning sensation. Gauze dressings are applied and changed until the bleeding subsides and an antibiotic ointment is applied to the treated areas. The physician may use warm air from a hair dryer to control the final bleeding and help the formation of a crust. Some physicians bandage the face after dermabrasion; others do not.

The same technique is used when the operation is performed under general anesthesia, except that the skin is not injected or sprayed. After the office procedure, the patients rest and then are sent home. Hospitalized patients return to their room.

After the Operation

Postoperative treatment consists of medication to ease pain, if necessary; antibiotics; and medication for sleeping. If a face bandage was applied, it is removed after 24 hours.

The skin is moist and may ooze a yellowish serum which, within 24 to 36 hours, develops into a firm crust. The face swells—the greater the area that has been abraded, the greater the swelling will be. Sometimes the eyes are swollen almost shut the day after the operation. When the planing has been done near the mouth, the resulting crust makes it difficult to open the mouth, and patients may need to stay on a liquid diet for a few days. In most cases the swelling begins to decrease by the third postoperative day and the patient feels more comfortable.

The daily use of a bland cream, ointment, or oil is generally recommended to keep the crusts soft. Some doctors prescribe warm-water soaks, begun five days after the operation, to further soften them. The crusts separate from the underlying skin in seven to ten days, depending on the age of the patient and the depth of the abrasion. Hair should not be washed and men should not shave until the crusts have fallen off.

The skin that appears as the crusts peel off ranges from light to bright pink. At its first appearance, the new skin is better than the final result because it is still swollen, and the swelling masks any small lines or scars that are still present. After about three to four weeks the skin generally settles. This stage can be a time of disappointment for people who had the notion that their skin was going to take a giant leap back through time and come up firm and smooth like a baby's cheek. But those with more realistic expectations are often very pleased. The pinkness fades gradually after a month or a month and a half, although it can continue up to three months.

Most patients are able to resume their usual activities after two weeks, although older people may need an additional week. The delay in getting back into the world is mainly caused by self-consciousness rather than by any discomfort. If only a spot abrasion was done and the patients do not mind the appearance of the scab, they can return to work or school the following day.

Follow-Up

Very few follow-up visits are required. The surgeon may want to see the patient after the crust has gone and then perhaps for an occasional checkup over the next several months. The patient is instructed in the care of the skin by the surgeon.

Caring for the New Skin

How well the new skin holds up depends to a degree on the care the patient gives it. The skin will be tender and easily irritated for several months, until it has a chance to regenerate and regain its normal pigment and color. Some physicians feel that irregular pigmentation occurring in a newly abraded skin is associated with excessive exposure to the sun. It is essential, therefore, to avoid exposure to direct or reflected sunlight for at least two to four months following the treatment. A good quality sunscreen cream must be used during this period, or longer. The skin should be kept scrupulously clean and treated nightly with a soothing ointment or cream. Ordinary cosmetics may be used as soon as the abraded areas have healed, but strong soaps and medicated cosmetics should be avoided.

Complications

Infection following dermabrasion is rare because of the rich blood supply to the face. The most common reaction is the formation of tiny milia (whiteheads) during the third or fourth week after surgery. They occur in about 40 percent of patients and sometimes disappear spontaneously, helped along by cleansing the area with a washcloth. If not, they are easily removed without scarring either by being pierced and expressed with a whitehead remover, or by electrodesiccation (using an electric needle to destroy tissue).

Alteration of the pigment in the skin occurs in all patients for several weeks. At first, the skin loses pigment and is bright pink. It takes about six weeks for the skin to return to normal, although some skins may take up to three months or longer. A postinflammatory darkening of the skin (hyperpigmentation) occurs in a significant percentage of people even without exposure to the sun. This darkening may persist for months or years before the face returns to a uniform color, and it must be protected by special sunscreens. Less often, loss of pigment occurs in the abraded areas (hypopigmentation). It is generally irreversible but can be camouflaged by makeup.

Fees

The fees for a full face dermabrasion range from $700 to $2,000. Partial or spot dermabrasion costs from $500 upwards, depending on how much is done. For general anesthesia, the anesthetist's fee may range from $200 to 20 percent of the surgeon's fee.

In some instances when a surgeon knows in advance that more than one dermabrasion will be necessary, the fee for succeeding operations is reduced. Amy J. has had three dermabrasions over the last two and a half years for moderately severe acne scars. She reports that her physician has a special fee arrangement in such situations.

One Patient's Experience

It would take close examination by a trained eye to see the remains of acne scars on Amy's face. She has large-pored skin with minor irregularities; her skin is neither bad nor lovely. Amy, who is 28 years old and a chief administrator in a large office, says:

It never occurred to me that I wouldn't have to carry an acne-scarred face for the rest of my life....

I was always miserable about my skin. I had bad acne in my teens and early twenties. It finally quieted down, but it left its mark. Makeup never concealed the pits and scars and I was always terribly self-conscious about it. I was delighted when I learned that maybe it could be improved.

The physician who treated Amy performed the dermabrasion in the office. He told her that she would probably need three operations to achieve optimum results. Amy recalls the first:

It was done on a Friday, which gave me two whole weekends to recover, and I was able to go back to my office ten days later, missing just six working days. I must say I was looking awfully pink and blotchy, but otherwise not too bad. The operation itself was easier than I had expected. The freezing process before the abrading began was uncomfortable, but I don't recall minding the rest of it particularly. The bandages were left on

150

for 24 hours and I couldn't eat during that time—just fluids through a straw. The bandages don't allow for chewing, and, besides that, my face was stiff as a plaster mask from the crusting.

But the worst shock, as I remember, was when the bandages came off. How can I describe what my face looked like? ... Raw meat, maybe ... a horror. I told the doctor that I thought he made a mistake not to let the patient see how she looks before she is bandaged, so she's better prepared for the vision that's waiting behind the bandage.

But outside of the trauma of looking at myself, there was no particular pain after that. I did all the things I was told to with warm-water soaks and creams, and finally all the crusts came off. My face was sort of mottled and was a symphony in pinks—from light pink to bright pink— like a severe sunburn. This gradually faded but it took a good six weeks.

My skin looked unbelievably smooth for the first couple of months while it was still swollen, but it settled down after a while and was less smooth, but better than before the dermabrasion. The doctor told me this would happen so I was prepared. The next two dermabrasions each brought some additional improvement, so while I can't say I've had perfect results, I think it's fair to say it's 75 or maybe 80 percent better than it was, which I feel made the dermabrasion worthwhile.

Chemical Face Peel

Chemical skin peeling, also known as chemosurgery and chemabrasion, is a procedure in which a caustic chemical solution is applied to the skin to remove the outer layer (epidermis) and the upper layers of the tier of fibrous, connective tissue that are just below it (dermis). What happens, in effect, is a controlled second-degree burn caused by the application of a chemical solution. After the application of the chemicals, the cauterized tissue remains in place while the new skin is formed beneath it, whereas in dermabrasion the top layers of the skin are removed immediately.

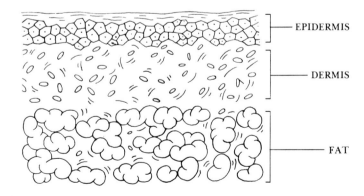

EPIDERMIS

DERMIS

FAT

CROSS SECTION OF SKIN

The chemical peel is generally most effective in improving or eradicating shallow forehead wrinkles, creases, facial pigmentations, minor skin blemishes, cheek wrinkles, and the fine lines about the eyes and lips. It is useless for facial sags and pouches, which respond only to face lifting. In conjunction with a face lift, however, it can do wonders in restoring a youthful appearance. Small areas of the face, such as around the lips or the forehead, may be done at the same time as a face lift, but an entire face peel must be performed separately, well after the face has recovered from the trauma of the face lift operation.

The results of a successful chemical peel can be a triumph—the skin appears firmer and smoother—but the chemicals used are powerful, and in the wrong hands the procedure can be a disaster for the patient, both physically and aesthetically. It should be done only by a qualified plastic surgeon or dermatologist who understands how to apply the chemicals judiciously and the types of skin that will react favorably to them. The ignorant use of these strong chemicals by unknowing lay operators has caused great damage to people's bodies and health. Because the effects of the chemicals can be unpredictable in some instances, the chemical face peel has not yet earned the unqualified approval of all physicians, although it has many enthusiastic champions.

How It Began

It is a curious historical fact that the areas of medicine we now consider leading specialties—diseases of the eye, ear, skin, nose and throat—were until around 1800 in the hands of quacks, literally thrust there by the medical profession. We might well agonize over the plight of the unfortunate patient in the 18th Century who had a serious eye or ear problem. When a distinguished British physician founded a hospital in London in 1805 for the exclusive care of eye patients, he apologized to his colleagues for invading the field presided over by quacks. Similarly, the popularity of the skin peel with chemicals first gained notoriety through its use by lay operators. By 1960, however, it had found a place in the literature of plastic surgery and it has been refined over the years to its present place in the armamentarium of ethical medical practitioners.

Patient Selection

Not everyone is a suitable candidate for a chemical face peel. Its use is contraindicated in the presence of a number of diseases, particularly kidney disease or malfunctioning kidneys, because the most frequently used basic agent for the chemical peel is phenol (carbolic acid), which is absorbed in part through the skin into the circulation of the body and may be harmful to the kidneys. In spite of its toxic qualities, it remains the chemical of choice among most surgeons for its effectiveness and relative predictability when properly used.

Not understood by the lay operator is the fact that phenol is made more dangerous rather than less so by being diluted. The stronger the acid, the more quickly it creates a barrier when it touches the skin, which prevents the chemical from seeping through the dermis and into the blood. Uninformed lay operators mistakenly believe that they are providing safety by diluting the acids, when in fact they are doing just the opposite. The slower the burn, the greater the chances for systemic absorption.

People with fair skins are better prospects for chemabrasion than those with darker complexions. The olive-skinned patients may show a noticeable contrast between the treated and untreated areas, and the final skin color may be blotchy. Black-skinned people are generally not good risks because of their color and because of their tendency to form keloids. Also contraindicated are persons with skin that has had radiation treatment or has been burned. Such skin lacks regenerating cells and will not heal well. The thin-skinned sections of the body, such as the neck, chest, arms, and back of the hands are also poorly supplied with regenerative tissue and should not be treated because of the danger of scarring.

Chemabrasion is usually confined only to the skin of the face. If the surgeon has any suspicion about how the skin will react to the chemical peel, he will apply the phenol to a small test area in front of or behind the ear near the hairline. If there is no scarring after two to four weeks, he may feel it is safe to proceed with the entire face. This method is the only one the surgeon has to predict the effect of the chemical on the patient's skin.

Before the Operation

The usual preoperative photographs may be taken. The chemical peel is an uncomfortable experience and the aftermath, with the crusting of the face, can be an ordeal psychologically if not physically. As with dermabrasion, patients may be housebound for ten days or so because of their appearance, and those people who live alone may need to enlist the aid of friends or family to take care of their errands.

The chemical peel may be an office procedure if only a small part of the face is being treated, but most surgeons prefer to do the full face in a hospital. The usual hospital stay is three days. Patients are admitted the day before and a physical examination and laboratory tests are done. The face and hair are washed that evening with an antibacterial soap and the face is washed thoroughly again the morning of the surgery. No anesthesia is used for the chemical peel, but the patient is premedicated.

The Operation

After the patient is on the operating table, the face is thoroughly cleansed with a small amount of ether so there will be no skin oils or remaining soap to interfere with the even penetration of the phenol. The phenol is combined with other chemicals and ingredients that enhance its action and act as a buffer. This solution is applied with a brush or a cotton-tipped applicator stick. Patients generally feel a momentary stinging or burning sensation that passes rapidly and is replaced by anesthesia. The skin is gently stretched as the application is made so that the wrinkles will be flattened and the fluid will coat the skin evenly. Almost immediately after the chemical solution is applied, the skin turns frosty white (blanches) for two or three minutes. It then becomes swollen and turns dark red.

The procedure is done in sections—first the forehead and upper lids, then around the eyes, along the nose and upper lip (the nostrils are plugged with cotton to prevent the patient from inhaling the fumes of the phenol), the right cheek, the left cheek, and so on. The application of the solution is carried into the hairline and just below the jawline to avoid a demarcation between the treated and untreated skin and to the very border of the lips since a band of untreated skin here would be unattractive. The surgeon works very slowly, taking at least half an hour so that the phenol enters the system gradually.

Surgeons sometimes apply two or three layers of waterproof adhesive tape to each section of the face as it is treated, leaving only the eyes, nostrils, and lips exposed. This tape mask intensifies the action of the chemical, causing a deeper peel with more lasting results, but adds greatly to the discomfort of the patient. After the application of the tape mask—or sometimes even without it—the burning sensation may return and last for an hour or two, requiring further sedation. The surgeon's decision whether to use the "lighter" treatment without the adhesive dressing or the "deeper" one with the adhesive is influenced by the type and condition of the skin. A thin, finely textured skin with light wrinkling may not require taping, but a severely weather-beaten face would do well to have it.

After
the Operation

Bed rest is recommended for at least the first 24 hours. If the lips were done, a liquid diet sipped through a straw is desirable. Chewing and talking should be kept to a minimum for the first few days. The patient may need additional medication to be comfortable. The skin begins to swell immediately after the operation and in a few hours it turns brown and exudes a clear fluid. The eyelids may swell shut. Intense swelling of the face persists for three to four days. Ice packs to the eyes and keeping the head elevated can be helpful.

154

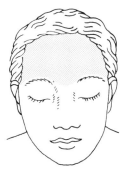 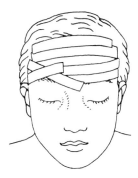

In the chemical peel, a chemical solution is first applied to the forehead. For a deeper peel, the treated skin is covered with layers of adhesive tape.

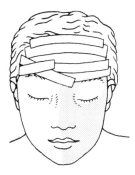 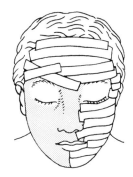

The face is treated in small sections and the chemical solution is applied slowly. The eyelids, nostrils, and lips are left exposed. Treating the entire face takes about 30 minutes.

The tape mask remains for 48 hours and is then removed.

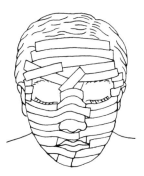

By about the third day, a dry crust begins to form and the swelling begins to subside. At this time there can be some itching and discomfort. As the crust loosens, serum oozes from beneath the cracks. The first crust separation begins from the fifth to the seventh day after the operation. Starting about the fifth day, patients are generally instructed to apply a liberal coating of bland cold cream, or a salve of the surgeon's choice. Some sur-

155

geons recommend Crisco. The crust continues to slough off, and generally by the tenth to the fourteenth day, the crust has completely crumbled away, leaving a clear, firm, deep-pink skin.

The postoperative procedure when the skin has been taped differs somewhat. Forty-eight hours after the application of the chemical peel, the adhesive mask is removed. This can be painful and the patient will require sedation in advance. With the mask off, the skin is raw and moist. It is sprinkled generously with an iodide powder that produces a white pebbly coating. The application is repeated as often as needed to maintain a dry surface—perhaps two or three times a day for three days. The powder mask is removed about a week later. To facilitate its removal, the patient applies a cream or Crisco the day before.

The moment the mask is removed is generally a most exciting one for the patient. The skin may be a deep crimson, but it will look soft and smooth, although the face will feel tight on the slightest movement. The skin is still swollen and residual wrinkles, which may appear later, are not yet in evidence. However, surgeons always warn their patients that some of the fine lines may reappear. The realistic patient whose hopes are not too high will not be disappointed when the skin recovers from the punishment it has taken and settles down. There seem to be enough satisfactory results from the chemical peel to encourage people to undergo the rigors of the operation. Those patients who expect that every wrinkle and line will be erased are indulging themselves in fantasy and wishful thinking. A skin that has weathered 40 or 50 years or more can be improved but not magically transformed.

Caring for the
New Skin

Once the crusts are completely gone, the face can be washed with mild soap and water. The skin should be treated with a gentle cream or moisturizer. Regular makeup may be applied after two or three weeks. The skin feels rather tight at first, but gradually relaxes.

The intense crimson of the skin fades within a short time, but the skin may remain excessively pink for from six to eight weeks or even longer. The most important consideration in the care of the new skin is the avoidance of sunlight for about six months. Irregular pigmentation of the skin can result from overexposure or even spontaneously. Avoidance of direct sun, a broad-brimmed hat, and the use of a good sunscreen preparation are cardinal rules to be observed in the care and protection of the new skin.

Chemical peeling may be repeated cautiously. There is no general agreement among surgeons about the ideal time interval between treatments. Some feel that limited areas can be retreated in a matter of weeks and the whole face in a few months; others recommend a rest period between chemical peels of from 12 to 18 months.

The most common problem following chemical peeling is the difference in skin color between the treated and untreated areas. This disparity is less likely to occur in persons with light hair, blue eyes, and light skin. Dark-skinned people sometimes develop dark patches of pigmentation (hyperpigmentation) following chemical peel. The patches may fade spontaneously after months or even years. Creams or lotions containing bleaching agents may be of some help. Occasionally loss of pigment (hypopigmentation) takes place. It is generally permanent and can be concealed by makeup.

Tiny milia (whiteheads), which sometimes appear in the treated areas, may disappear spontaneously after a few weeks, helped by the abrasive action of a washcloth. If not, they can be pierced and expressed with a whitehead remover or removed by electrodesiccation.

Hypertrophic scars (heavy raised scars) are always a threat and a danger, but careful selection of patients, pretesting, and skilled application of the chemical solution by an experienced plastic surgeon or dermatologist militate against this complication. Chemical peeling on the neck and arms is avoided. Occasionally the neck is done lightly with a buffered chemical solution, but no area below the neck is ever touched.

Another complication of the chemical peel, as with all aesthetic surgery, is the result not consistent with what the patient had in mind. The skin generally looks smoother and firmer and more youthful, but every line cannot be eradicated and a large-pored skin will remain a large-pored skin. How long the skin retains its tight new look depends in part on the patient's condition and lifestyle. Good skin care, avoidance of sun, and a stable body weight will help to preserve it. But the new skin is living tissue and will gradually age, just as it did before.

Complications

Full face chemical peel ranges from $750 to $2,000. Partial chemabrasion is less.

Fees

Virginia W., a 44-year-old housewife and the mother of three teenage children, is a pleasant looking woman with brown hair, blue eyes, and a fairly smooth, fine-textured skin. She wears little makeup. A few years earlier, a cyst had been clumsily removed from her right cheek, and she was left with a disfiguring scar, which was subsequently treated by dermabrasion. The result was unsatisfactory. The plastic surgeon she consulted thought she

One Patient's Response

would benefit most from a chemical face peel because she also had a few lines and some scattered areas of pigmentation. Two months after the operation she was asked how she felt about it.

I was very eager for the operation. The scar on my cheek looked like a vaccination that ended up in the wrong place and I was never good at covering it up. I never liked using a lot of makeup. It had reached the point where the only thing I could see when I looked in the mirror was the scar on my cheek.

I have to admit that I felt guilty about wanting to have it done—I still do. After all, it's an expensive business and I was afraid that my husband, and the children particularly, would resent my being so self-indulgent. There are so many things they ask for that we have to tell them we can't afford. But they were very sweet and generous and they all encouraged me.

The operation itself was unpleasant but not intolerable. After the solution was applied there was a burning sensation and then no feeling. But then your face turns red and then brown and it puffs and it weeps—it's a mess. No matter how your surgeon tries to prepare you for the way you're going to look, you can't quite believe it will be that bad. But it's worse. I left the hospital the day after the operation with my face swathed in a scarf. That was one time I didn't want to be seen.

The first few days were uncomfortable. My face was stiff and I couldn't eat or talk. The surgeon had warned me that there would be some itching on the third or fourth day. Instead of itching, I had the most intense pain I've ever experienced. It was a burning agony and it lasted for more than a day. Ice compresses eased it a little and some medication helped, but it was a bad time. I wonder if the surgeon knew there was going to be that much pain or if it's unusual....

After that, I got along very well, I think. By ten days after the operation, the crust was all off and my face was smooth and tight but flaming red. It's been fading right along and I'm almost back to my normal color. My skin is much smoother and nicer than it was before and the scar on my cheek is almost unnoticeable. I'm glad I did it, of course, and even more glad that I don't have to do it again.

The children are the best part of it. They seem to get more pleasure out of the way I look than I do. I think perhaps the scar bothered them too.

Liquid-Silicone Injections

A great deal has been written about the use and misuse of liquid silicone over the last number of years. It first attracted attention in the mid-1950s, with reports of an unidentified injectable liquid that was being used in Europe and in the Orient as a fat substitute for filling out depressions in the contour of soft tissues, particularly for breast augmentation. For centuries medical men had dreamed of just such a substance—one that would fill a long list of criteria ranging from being nontoxic and noncarcinogenic to being simple to prepare and sterilize. The product, which was finally identified by the formidable name of dimethylpolysiloxane fluid, a silicone compound, gave promise of fulfilling this dream. Injections of liquid silicone have been found effective in plumping up certain facial lines and wrinkles, in rounding out chins that were a tiny bit too small, in creating the illusion of high cheekbones where none had existed, in filling out depressions in the bridge or tip of the nose left by inept nasal reconstructions, in improving certain types of depressed scars, in restoring the contour of faces wasted with disease, and more.

Silicone is an extraordinary product. In its solid form, it has branched out from its thousands of industrial uses to become part of the armamentarium of plastic surgeons as bone and cartilage substitutes. Only specially manufactured, medical grade silicone products are used by the medical profession. It ranges in consistency from watery liquids, oils, and thick honeylike gels to sponge, foam, and hard silicone rubber. It is an inert, unchanging material unaffected by years of exposure to the elements. The medical grade fluids do not evaporate or turn gummy. The silicone rubber does not deteriorate.

Controversy over Liquid Silicone

No one questions the value of solid silicone as chin, ear, nose, and other subcutaneous implants, or the value of the breast implant of translucent silicone gel contained in a seamless, thin-walled silicone envelope. These implants have been a boon to thousands of physicians and hundreds of thousands of patients. It is the liquid silicone that has been under scrutiny since the middle 1960s and its use is now highly controversial.

At that time, Dow Corning, its principal manufacturer, became concerned over reports of unfortunate aftereffects of silicone injections. Its very advantages proved its undoing. The fact that it could be injected in a face or a breast to increase tissue volume, thereby avoiding a surgical procedure requiring an implant, made it a most attractive technique to the lay public and to physicians. Too many physicians, unskilled and inexperienced in its use, were using it improperly. When liquid silicone is injected in too large an amount, it drifts to undesired locations, masquerading as cysts or tumors. Once in the body, it is mostly irretrievable—it cannot be totally removed. Limited dosage had to be rigidly observed, yet it was impossible to police the physicians who were using it incorrectly.

Dow Corning voluntarily listed liquid silicone with the Food and Drug Administration, which meant that the silicone was no longer an implant material but was classified as a drug. The company then made the medically pure, injectable silicone available to seven plastic surgeons and one dermatologist throughout the United States for clinical study. However, there are other physicians in possession of the medically pure liquid silicone who are skilled in its use.

Pros and Cons of Liquid-Silicone Injections

All ethical physicians are in complete agreement about the unsuitability of liquid-silicone injections for breast augmentation. There is also total agreement about the value of injectable silicone for two rare and little-understood diseases—facial hemiatrophy and facial lipodystrophy. They are similar to one another. In the first, there is a wasting away of the skin, underlying facial muscles and, in some instances, bone and cartilage on one side of the face. In facial lipodystrophy, the wasting extends to the entire face and neck, and often to the upper part of the arms and torso. Injections of liquid silicone beneath the skin produce a dramatic improvement in the appearance of the patients and is without equal in the treatment of the two diseases. Follow-up examinations over a number of years have shown no migration of the silicone and no lessening in improvement.

At this point, the agreement about injectable silicone ends. There is no unanimity of opinion—even among the eight investigators. Some disapprove of it, others are ambivalent, and a few are highly enthusiastic. This last group have used it with great success. Unequivocally they declare it "safe and effective."

Method of Injection

The champions of liquid-silicone injections maintain that the problem with it lies in improper administration. It must be injected a droplet at a time beneath the deepest stratum of the skin. The liquid is the consistency of mineral oil and a very fine needle is necessary, so it requires great patience on the part of the physician. A small amount of liquid silicone—perhaps only 20 drops—is injected, at well-spaced intervals (once or twice a month), and it may take a number of sessions to fill out one small line or wrinkle.

The injections are given with the patient lying down quietly. The skin is cleansed. Local anesthesia is rarely used because of the danger of distorting the tissues and thus misleading the surgeon about the amount of silicone needed. The injections are closely spaced along the wrinkle. Immediately following the injection, the physician massages the area to make sure the droplets spread evenly. Some physicians have a hand-held vibrating machine for this purpose. After each droplet is deposited in the skin, it gradually becomes surrounded by a tiny capsule of fibrous tissue, which is how the body reacts to anything that enters its tissues. Thus when the silicone is distributed evenly—instead of being pushed into a limited area—and enough time is

160

Liquid silicone can be effective in plumping up certain facial lines and wrinkles when used properly by an experienced physician.

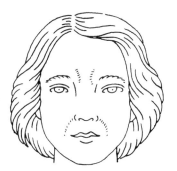

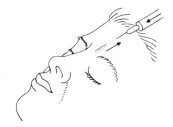 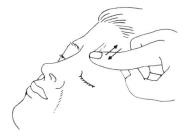

The silicone is injected into the wrinkle in tiny quantities. Pressure is applied to the injected site to spread the liquid silicone evenly underneath the skin.

allowed between injections, the droplets are virtually trapped in place by a lacing of fibrous tissues that keeps them from migrating into surrounding tissues.

Pain or discomfort after the injection is rare. There may be some swelling and, if a vein was punctured, some black and blue discoloration, but these are self-limiting. Occasionally, because of the progression of wrinkling, booster shots may be required at intervals of several months after the final result has been achieved.

Indiscriminate use of nonmedical grade injectable silicone can only be condemned. When injected in impure or contaminated forms, the silicone can cause chronic inflammation. Medically pure silicone in the hands of skillful physicians, trained in its use and familiar with its idiosyncrasies, has proved of value in treating some of the aesthetically unwelcome signs of aging.

Conclusions

At present, liquid silicone is still considered an experimental drug, and Dow Corning is not pursuing its application with the Food and Drug Administration for permission to market the substance, which will tend to keep it out of the hands of people untrained in its use. The American Society of Plastic and Reconstructive Surgeons is supporting an effort to organize a program in which 25 plastic surgeons in various parts of the country will have the liquid silicone available for special cases of congenital or traumatic facial deformities for which there is no other satisfactory treatment.

Information about names of physicians who use liquid-silicone therapy may be obtained by writing the American Society of Plastic and Reconstructive Surgeons, Inc., 29 East Madison Street, Chicago, Illinois 60602, or the American Academy of Dermatology, 820 Davis Street, Evanston, Illinois 60201.

Fees

Fees vary widely. In one office, the physician charges $20 for the liquid silicone and $40 for administering it—per session. The number of sessions required depends on the extent of the area to be treated.

Correction of Scars

Scars that result from injury or accident can be as psychologically damaging as they are aesthetically unpleasing. Plastic surgery can often improve the appearance of an unsightly scar by replacing it with a finer, less conspicuous one. However, it cannot perform sleight of hand, like the black-caped magician with a deck of playing cards, waving away all traces of it. Patients must understand this if they are not to be disappointed. The final results of scar correction will depend on a number of factors: the age of the patient, the location of the scar, the amount of skin loss, the age of the scar and its cause, and the general health of the patient. In some cases, surgery for the correction of scars may need to be followed by dermabrasion or chemical peeling to achieve an optimum result.

Treating scars in children is less satisfactory than in adults. Children heal faster than adults but not as well. Increased skin elasticity, increased skin tension, and the elements of growth present in the young militate against the final result. Scars in children tend to become wide and overgrown (hypertrophic), remain pink longer, and flatten more slowly.

The surgeon plans the correction of the scar with great care, paying particular attention to the depth and width of the scar, and the direction of the muscle layers of the skin. If there is sufficient skin, the scar may be excised and the wound closed without tension. A wide and irregular scar may require a series of operations, each one removing a part of the old scar until only a fine line remains of the last scar. When there is not sufficient skin to be drawn together without tension, a skin graft from the patient's own body must be provided.

Some skins have a tendency to heal with a heavy weltlike overgrowth called a keloid or hypertrophic scar. A hypertrophic scar usually stops growing after about three months and then slowly softens. The keloid, in contrast, may remain red and raised during the patient's lifetime and even increase in size. Cortisone injections and x-ray therapy are used when indicated to treat both types of scars.

In most instances, scar correction should be delayed until the scar has had time to mature. The healing process is considered complete when the scar has become soft and white, which may take as long as six months. Waiting out this period will often eliminate the need for scar revision or at least minimize the operation. Time itself frequently has a way of changing a red raised scar to a flat white one and reducing the itching and burning that sometimes accompany the scars. There are some emergency situations, however, where scar revisions may be undertaken earlier, as with scars resulting from burns. This type of scar contracts and restricts motion. Correction may require several plastic procedures involving skin grafting.

Most scar revisions of limited extent can be performed under local anesthesia. Extensive surgery involving skin grafts or flaps requires general anesthesia in a hospital.

Not all scar corrections are completely successful, but there are many results that are almost a major miracle, where not only the patient's face is restored but the patient's spirit as well. Eleanor N. is a perfect example and her appearance today represents a triumph for the art of plastic surgery. She is an attractive young lady in her middle thirties. One might notice a slight unevenness in the skin on her chin which could have been the result of adolescent acne but nothing worthy of a question or second glance.

Six years earlier, Eleanor had been vacationing in Australia with some friends. The car in which they had been touring was involved in a bad accident near a small village miles away from any large city. She had been sitting in the front seat of the car. The windshield was shattered and her face was cut. She was not aware of the extent of her injuries at that moment. She was taken to a nearby hospital and for three hours the local doctor stitched her face together as well as he could.

I'm not going to describe how I looked, except to tell you that there wasn't a square inch of my face from my eyebrows to my chin that wasn't slashed or torn. As a matter of fact, pieces of glass kept surfacing up until four years after the accident.

I returned home the following month—with half a dozen plastic caps on my front teeth to cover the broken teeth—and started to make the rounds of plastic surgeons. I was told I would have to wait six to nine months before any repairs could be started in order to give the swelling time to go down and the scars to stabilize.

Eleanor is an extremely controlled young woman who is given to understatement, but one doesn't need much imagination to sense the agony of that period. Outside of seeing a few close friends, she had no social life. Her place of employment transferred her to an office job away from the public.

Children on buses would cry from fear when they saw me. My face was a mass of red, raised jagged scars. My mouth was twisted into a permanent grimace and I couldn't close my lips because of the scar tissue. I avoided mirrors and people. I don't want to think about what went on in my head at that time, but I was afraid to go too close to a window for fear that I might not be able to control my impulses.

Then I started seeing plastic surgeons. One said a series of eight or nine operations with local anesthesia; another said three or four under general ... and I became more and more confused. Was there a right way and a wrong way? Then I was referred to still another plastic surgeon and everything came together. He made no promises. He said I would need a series of operations and treatment would take years. He couldn't guarantee results, but he felt he could effect an improvement.

Seven operations were performed on my face over the next four years. They were all done in the operating room in his office under local anesthesia. Following the first few operations, I was bandaged like a mummy for two to four days each time. I could scarcely speak and had to be on a liquid diet. He started with the very worst places on my chin which had ledges of scar tissue. He excised the scar tissue—fortunately there was enough skin to stretch. He had to do only one skin graft on the chin with a small piece of skin taken from in front of my ear, and the scar doesn't even show.

I never would have believed a few years back that a face as mutilated as mine could ever be restored to anything resembling normalcy—or that I would reach the point where that wretched period of anxiety and self-consciousness would be a closed chapter in my life.

Fees

Fees for scar revisions vary widely, depending on the size and location of the scars and the complexity of the operation. The fee for the excision of a facial scar can range from $250 to $1,500 and can go upwards for a complicated scar or scars that involve one of the features of the face.

Superficial Skin Lesions

The majority of superficial skin lesions such as moles, warts, or "spiders" (clusters of tiny capillary blood vessels in the superficial skin) can be treated by a dermatologist in the office. Minor cosmetic surgery is frequently performed with an electric needle

164

by a process called electrodesiccation, which uses high-frequency electric current that destroys tissue. Since there can be some pain involved if the lesion is large, local anesthesia may be injected or sprayed. A scab results from electrodesiccation, which falls off after a few days. A scar may or may not result, depending on how much tissue was destroyed.

There are two types of keratoses—seborrheic and actinic. An experienced dermatologist can generally distinguish between the two, although it is not always an easy diagnosis to make. **Keratosis**

Seborrheic keratosis is a common lesion often appearing in large numbers, especially on the trunk, face, neck, scalp, and arms of middle-aged or older persons. The lesions are sharply circumscribed, cauliflowerlike, raised, have scaly patches, and range in color from brown to black. They are described as having a "stuck-on appearance." Their only significance is as a cosmetic disfigurement. They may be removed by scraping with a curette or by electrodesiccation. Sometimes they are treated by nonsurgical means such as freezing or the application of a medication with a selective corrosive action.

Actinic keratosis, also known as solar or senile keratosis, develops in areas of chronic exposure to sunlight. Fair-skinned persons are more prone to develop them. The lesions are small and flat or slightly raised and grayish or brownish in color, and may be rough or covered with scales. They are often numerous in elderly people with weather-beaten skin. These lesions are regarded as precancerous and should be carefully watched by a physician. It is essential that persons whose skins demonstrate these changes avoid overexposure to sunlight. They are removed by the same methods used for the seborrheic keratoses.

Warts are infections caused by a virus. Scratching one with a comb, fingernail, or razor may spread the infection. There are a variety of ways of treating warts, but no one way can be said to be 100 percent effective in every case. Among the methods of treating them are electrodesiccation, curettage, application of acid, and freezing with liquid nitrogen or dry ice. **Warts**

The most common type of xanthoma is the soft, yellowish, slightly raised, velvety patch that appears on the eyelids, usually near the inner corners. A few people who develop them have heightened cholesterol with the risk of early atherosclerosis, but in many cases there is no metabolic disturbance and the xanthomas are purely an aesthetic problem. They are treated by **Xanthomas** excision, electrodesiccation, or applications of acid. Recurrence is common. The important thing is to look for possible causes.

Moles

Moles are pigmented lesions that can be flat or raised and may appear any place on the body. Every adult has at least a few moles and some may have hundreds. They may range in color from light yellowish brown to jet black. They can be the size of a pinhead or cover a large area of the body. They can be smooth or hairy. They can be benign or malignant and should be evaluated by a physician to determine in which category they belong. It is by no means practical or even justifiable to remove all moles. The decision requires expert judgment.

Excision is the accepted treatment for pigmented moles. A small excision will not require sutures. A biopsy is always done on a pigmented mole. A small light-colored mole which is aesthetically displeasing to its wearer may be removed by curettage or by electrodesiccation.

Spiders

Spiders, also known as telangiectasis, are a condition often acquired in later life, although they may appear before that. They are caused by abnormal capillaries that form in the superficial layer of the skin (epidermis), and are fed by a central small blood vessel. They may appear on the face or anywhere on the body. Treatment is rarely needed or requested for this condition. They can be destroyed by the application of dry ice or they may be sparked off by electrodesiccation. The action of the sparking is to cauterize the capillary, which cuts off the blood supply. After treatment, there is usually some redness and scab formation. The scab falls off in two or three days. Unfortunately, recurrences are common within a short time.

Tattoos

There are three kinds of tattoos—accidental, decorative, and medical. Accidental tattoos are formed by pigmented material being driven into the skin by an abrasive injury or an explosive force, such as road-dirt scrape or a gunpowder blast. Most of these lesions can be treated by vigorous brushing or dermabrasion to remove the small particles of pigment. Deeper specks may require a small curette or skin punch. Occasionally, hundreds of such excisions are necessary over a period of time.

Decorative tattoos may be removed by various surgical methods, but none is completely satisfactory because the tattoo pigment is deposited very deep into the skin and the removal of the tattoo usually results in a scar. Tattooing flesh-colored pigment over the original tattoo has not been satisfactory, since it is impossible to cover blue-black pigment with flesh-colored pigment. Also, tattooed areas contrast with tanned skin because tattooed areas will not tan. Skin planing is unsatisfactory; it must go so deep into the skin to reach the pigment that unsightly scars result. A degree of success is claimed by use of superficial dermabrasion and a procedure called salabrasion, in which table salt is rubbed over the tattooed area. Both of these procedures work on the principle that setting up an inflammatory reaction causes certain cells to pick up the tattoo pigment and work their way to the surface. However, a completely satisfactory method of tattoo removal has yet to be developed, and the person who has one removed generally has to decide whether he is willing to exchange the tattoo for the scar or defect that results from treatment.

Port-Wine Stains

This condition is a most difficult one to treat. Known technically as a hemangioma, this birthmark is produced by a congenital overgrowth of small blood vessels in the skin. Flat and bluish-red, they are commonly located on the head and neck and are usually on one side of the body, commonly ending at the midline of the face. Destruction of the tissue will replace the stain with even more objectionable scarring. Medical tattooing, which is tattooing with skin-colored pigment, is occasionally helpful, but it is difficult to match the pigment of the skin closely and the results leave something to be desired. The treatment is slow, tedious, and costly. When the stained area is small, it may be possible to do a skin graft. In rare cases, a dermabrasion is helpful. Generally, the best management for a port-wine stain is to use a specially designed masking cream to camouflage the lesion.

Rhinophyma

Rhinophyma is a bizarre and disfiguring overgrowth of the nose which is the end stage of a condition known as acne rosacea. It occurs mainly in men. It responds very well to surgical shaving of the thickened skin combined with dermabrasion. It is a hospital procedure requiring an overnight stay. The results of the surgery are dramatic. It may be done under general or local anesthesia.

Upper Lip Hair

While upper lip hair cannot by any means be considered an abnormality in women, a conspicuous growth of dark hair on the upper lip can be most distressing. It may be treated by bleaching, waxing, or electrolysis. When it is done properly, waxing of the upper lip is safe and does not inflict too much trauma on the skin. Electrolysis performed by an experienced operator is generally satisfactory. It should be understood, however, that it is not 100 percent permanent. Most of the hairs treated—but not all—are destroyed. Some will grow back and the treatment must be repeated.

167

DERMABRASION
FOR ACNE
SCARRING
Before

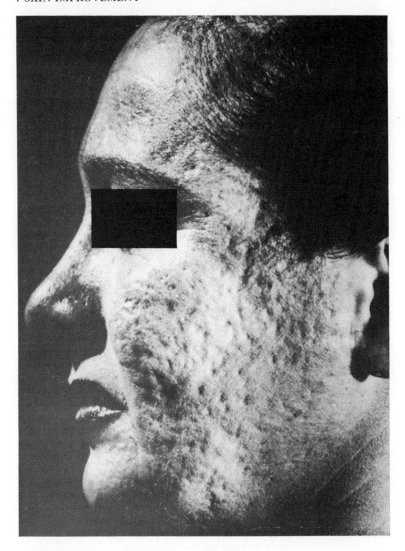

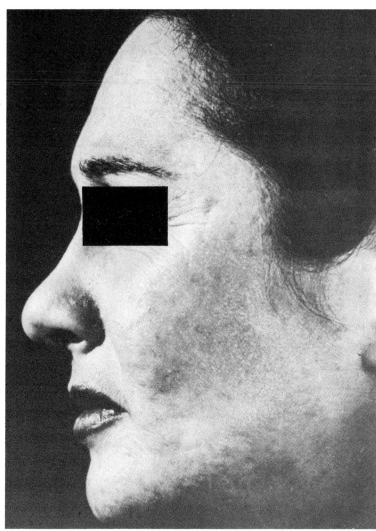

PHOTOGRAPHS COURTESY OF NORMAN ORENTREICH, M.D.

DERMABRASION
FOR
CORRECTION OF
WRINKLES
Before

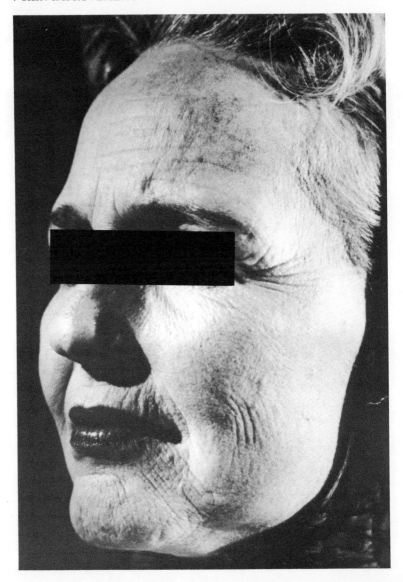

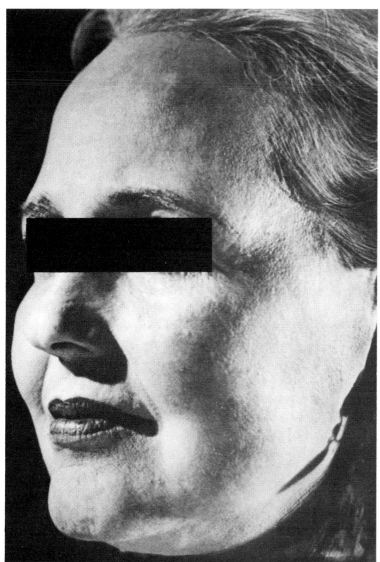

PHOTOGRAPHS COURTESY OF NORMAN ORENTREICH, M.D.

LIQUID–
SILICONE
INJECTIONS FOR
GLABELLA
Before

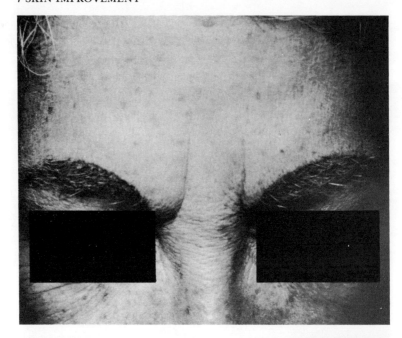

After

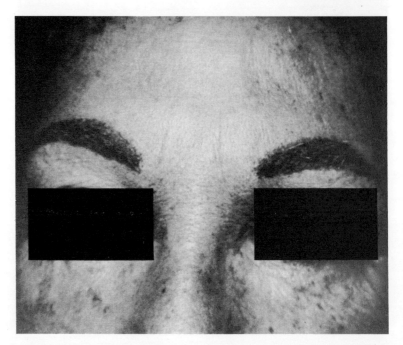

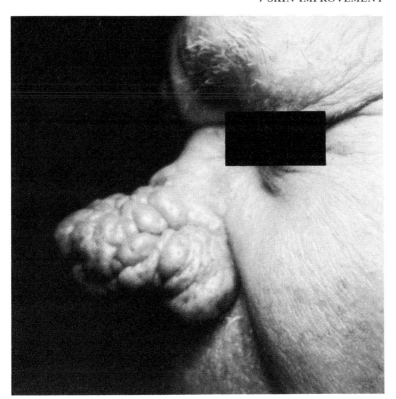

RHINOPHYMA
Before

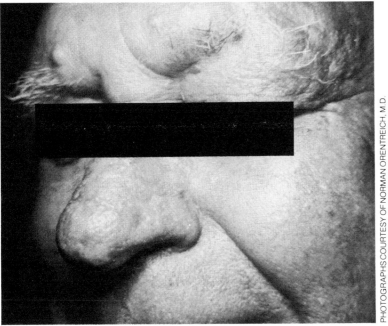

After

PHOTOGRAPHS COURTESY OF NORMAN ORENTREICH, M.D.

8

Hair Transplants

When Delilah severed Samson's seven tresses while he slept, she sheared him of his might and created a myth that has plagued the men of Western civilization since—to wit, a luxurious head of hair is synonymous with masculine potency, youth, and strength, whereas a bald or shaven scalp symbolizes loss of power and increasing age. For both men and women, plentiful hair connotes erotic allure at its peak. Conversely, in many cultures shorn hair is the sign of religious devotion, a monk or nun's deliberate abnegation of sexuality. Samson's hair, of course, grew back, but most men who lose hair today suffer from alopecia, called "male pattern baldness," an irreversible condition caused by a single unfriendly gene and normal male hormones.

Although hair loss is a normal physiological process (even without the hereditary factor, 100 percent of men and 85 percent of women lose hair as they grow older) and many ancient and modern figures of prominence were bald (for example, Cicero, Shakespeare, John D. Rockefeller, and Gerald Ford), few men suffer alopecia with equanimity. Even the two modern bald celebrities who slay women with their heavy sexual clout, Telly Savalas and Yul Brynner, provide little consolation for the two out of five men who find their hairlines creeping closer to the back of their scalp every year. Normal or not, alopecia is a trauma and the bald pate for most of us is a negative cultural image. "We're living in a hairy age," said one dermatologist. "Hair on the head and face is associated with a youthful image and sex appeal."

Until recently, there was no "cure" for alopecia. Hair-growing salves, shots of hormones into the scalp, diets, and massage devices have placed countless dollars into the pockets of quacks and very few hairs on anyone's head. Now, however, there is a simple, relatively painless, moderately priced surgical procedure, done with a local anesthetic in the office of the dermatologist, called a "hair transplant," in which small plugs of healthy, growing hair are removed from the back or sides of a balding patient's head and replanted in the hairless areas.

Miraculously, the hair begins to grow again in its new site just as it did before. After several procedures, when an appropriate number of plugs have been transplanted, the once bald patient has hair—his own hair, rooted in his own scalp, which he can wash, dye, pull, cut, brush, and braid.

The hair transplant operation, the least complicated of cosmetic surgical procedures, produces the fewest dissatisfied customers, when done correctly, and is used not only to create a new look of youth and vitality for men afflicted with normal male pattern baldness, but for patients of both sexes who have lost hair as a result of accidents such as burns or uncommon diseases that spontaneously destroy hair follicles and produce scars in their stead.

Causes
of Baldness

It is ironic that a man should consider his bald head a sign of lost virility, because it is precisely a man's maleness that helps to make him bald. In male pattern baldness, also called "androgenetic alopecia," hair loss occurs because the hair follicles in certain areas are genetically predisposed to develop a sensitivity to normal amounts of the male hormone, androgen, and to stop producing hair. Contrary to belief, it is the more "feminine" man, with more female hormones, who is less likely to become bald. Once a man is balding, there is only one known method to stop his hair from falling—to rid him of his masculinity altogether, or castrate him. Eunuchs are never bald. When they are given injections of male hormones, however, they will develop alopecia too, if they have the genetic predisposition to do so.

According to a common genetic theory, now under review by modern scientists, genetic inheritance is primarily responsible for the typical balding pattern experienced by 40 percent of the male population—that is, hair loss which leaves the top of the head and forehead bare while hair continues to sprout on the sides and back of the scalp. Male pattern baldness, it is often believed, is produced by a "sex-influenced gene," which is dominant in men and recessive in women. In other words, if a man inherits one unfriendly gene for baldness, either from his mother or his father, he will begin to lose hair at a genetically predetermined age. Women, on the other hand, must inherit two such genes before severe hair loss is a risk, and even with this double whammy they may never become completely bald, but may experience thinning of the hair or baldness in certain areas with advancing age.

Thus, a tendency to alopecia is a game of genetic Russian roulette. A man with a bald father will not necessarily become bald, since his father may have harbored only one gene for

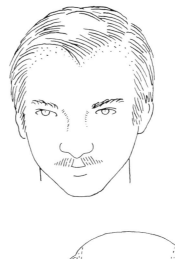

Inherited male pattern baldness begins with a receding hairline.

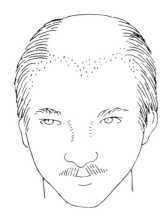

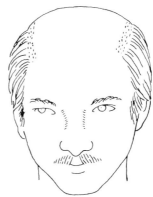

Gradually hair becomes thinner and more sparse on top. In the final stage hair grows only at the sides and back of the head.

baldness, and passed the other one to his son. A man who has a father and mother with full heads of hair may still inherit the fatal gene from his mother. All sons of bald women will be bald. Since the mother inherited two genes for baldness, she has to pass one of them to her sons. Baldness has been known to skip entire generations, but if there are no bald men on the father's side or the mother's side of the family, the children are probably safe from alopecia.

If a man inherits the gene for male pattern baldness, the hair follicles on the top of his head will eventually be obliterated by normal outputs of androgen, whereas the hair on the sides and back of his head probably will not. Aging, too, affects the inevitable process of hair loss, although dermatologists stress there is no *abnormal* age at which to begin losing hair if you are genetically predestined to do so. And hair loss may begin any time after puberty.

Although all races and ethnic groups have bald members, there is evidence that alopecia is less common among blacks than whites and least common among Asian peoples. If it is any comfort, some species of monkeys and birds develop male pattern baldness too.

The Physiological Process of Hair Loss

Hair itself is the proteinized end product of a growth process which begins below the surface of the skin in a tiny tunnel embedded in fat called the hair follicle. Cells in this dynamic structure reproduce rapidly, pushing a compact shaft composed of an elastic substance called keratin up and out of the skin. There are normally three phases to this growth process: the anagen, or active growing phase, the catagen, or regression phase, when the hair product is mature and the cellular activity necessary to produce it stops, and the telogen phase, when no growth occurs and the attachment of the hair to the base of the follicle becomes weaker and the hair falls out. In about three months after the hair falls, the growing phase begins again.

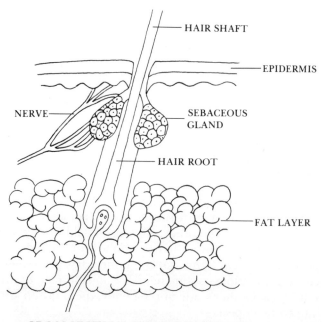

CROSS SECTION OF HAIR FOLLICLE

The three phases of growth fortunately affect different hairs throughout the scalp, so they are not all in the telogen phase at once. When hair loss begins, however, the follicles shrink after the mature hair falls, and the next generation of hair is thinner and lighter. When the atrophy of the follicle is complete, the hair diminishes to a fine fuzz, or there is no hair at all. Once the follicle ceases to produce, there is no way to regenerate it. The blood supply in the bald areas, however, remains the same, bringing a continual supply of oxygen and nutrients to the scalp.

Although typical male pattern baldness accounts for 95 percent of alopecia, there are other causes of balding as well. Surprisingly, perhaps, insufficient nourishment is not one of them. Although the hair quality of many species of mammals is strongly affected by diet, hair growth in human beings is little influenced by what they eat. Only in serious cases of malnourishment and vitamin deficiency is hair growth and color harmed. According to some dermatologists, severe nervous tension also fails to affect the hair.

Hair loss occurs as a result of burns, spontaneous scarring diseases, untreated diabetes, various malfunctions of the thyroid and pituitary glands, endocrine disorders, chemotherapy, radiation, and viral and fungous infections which affect the scalp. Often baldness is temporary and hair growth begins again when the condition that caused it is corrected. Temporary alopecia, for example, often occurs after pregnancy. Medication, too, can produce temporary baldness, and chemicals, used to enhance hair beauty, such as dyes and permanent-wave lotions, can strip the scalp of hair when incorrectly applied. Not to be underestimated is the balding effect of overbrushing and continuous pulling—from ponytails, tight braiding, chignons, curlers, bobby pins and combs—which is at first temporary, but can become permanent if constant trauma to an area is not alleviated.

Replacing Hair

Once the hair follicle atrophies, there is no way on earth to get it to bring forth hair. For centuries, however, men have refused to accept this universal truth and tried to reinstigate hair growth through a huge and bizarre assortment of cures. Thirty-five hundred years ago, an Egyptian papyrus was written recommending a regenerating salve, composed of fat of lion, fat of hippo, fat of crocodile, fat of cat, fat of serpent and ibex, mixed together to anoint the heads of bald Egyptians. Innumerable other useless remedies, from castor oil to hot beewax, have been recommended to the hairless throughout the ages.

In this century, when an American scientist conclusively connected male pattern baldness with the male hormone, doctors attempted to restore hair growth by injecting the bald scalp with female hormones. The fact is, only dangerous amounts of female hormones, enough to produce female secondary sex characteristics, can prevent further hair loss on the male scalp. "If a boy 20 years old is losing hair we could give him enough female hormones to stop it from falling out," one dermatologist said, "but he'd have to buy a bra, too." Injections of a cortico-steroid into the balding areas of scalps afflicted with a condition that produces patches of baldness, alopecia areata, however, are often useful.

Since it is impossible to revitalize a dead hair follicle, bald men and women must resort to illusion to recreate the youthful image of a full head of hair. Although wigs and hair pieces are good substitutes for real tresses, they have the disadvantage of slipping off at crucial moments. There are salons which specialize in hair weaving, a more stable form of the toupee; in this process, wefts of hair are woven into the customer's remaining strands and styled to cover bald areas. A surgical version of this procedure, hair implantation, is also becoming popular, but is strongly discouraged by dermatologists. In the hair implant, a Teflon-coated wire cable, something like the thread used for stringing beads, is woven in and out of the scalp with a needle. A hand-woven weft of hair, custom blended to match the customer's own in color and texture, is then attached to the loops of cable which remain outside the scalp. According to dermatologists, bacterial infections form easily at the fissures in the skin where the cable is implanted, and the body tends to reject the foreign substance. Also, the cable can be torn out of the scalp if enough pressure is applied.

Thus, the only safe, cosmetically effective method to give the illusion of hair growing on a bald head is the hair transplant, an operation developed by the American dermatologist Norman Orentreich, in 1959.

The Hair
Transplant

Plastic surgeons had previously attempted to camouflage baldness by grafting large hair-bearing flaps of flesh to bald areas, a complex and risky procedure. Orentreich discovered that it was easier, cosmetically more satisfying, and less dangerous to the patient to make the grafts smaller, and transfer tiny plugs of flesh containing hair follicles from their place of origin to the bald area, a procedure similar to re-sodding a lawn. He found that although the hair on the top of a balding man's head and the hair on the sides and back looked the same, it was physiologically different, and the follicles from the hair-bearing areas were no more affected by age and androgen when transplanted to the bald area than they were in their original site. The hair in the transplanted plugs, for some mysterious reason, continued to grow. "We could put these plugs in the palm of your hand and they'd still grow hair," said one dermatologist. The plugs will also grow in scar tissue, if it is not gangrenous. However, if alopecia should affect the hair on the back and sides of the head, the hair in the transplanted plugs will vanish too.

The transplant procedure, little changed since Orentreich first developed it, consists of punching out a small plug of flesh from a donor site, or a hair-bearing part of the scalp unthreatened by alopecia, with a metal punch and replacing it in a hole, excavated by the same punch, in the bald area of the head. The plugs taken from the donor sites are cleaned and trimmed of excess fat and hair in a sterile solution and the plugs taken from the bald areas are discarded. Then the doctor inserts the new plugs complete with hair follicles in the vacant spaces, stops bleeding, sometimes suturing the holes in the donor sites, bandages the head and sends the patient home. Crusts that soon form around the transplanted plugs heal and fall off in about two weeks.

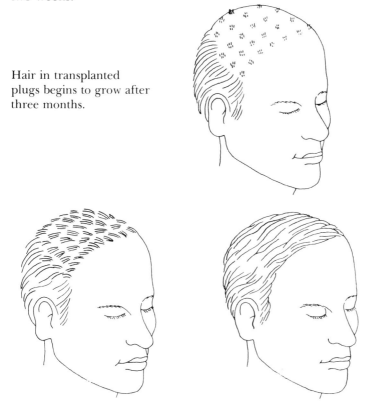

Hair in transplanted
plugs begins to grow after
three months.

The new hair continues to grow; good coverage is achieved after
several procedures.

The hair follicles, shaken by the trauma of surgery, go into a resting phase and the hair that was in them usually falls out. One hundred days later, however, the growing cycle begins again and the patient is ecstatic to see hair sprouting in what was once a barren soil. Due to the rich blood supply which surrounds the transplanted plugs, 99 percent "take," or establish a vascular relationship to their new bed, unless they are placed too closely together or the hair follicles in them were damaged during the surgical procedure. The operation is not complicated to perform. Many large offices, specializing in transplants, train registered nurses to do part of the job under a doctor's supervision. This does not mean, however, that *anyone* can do a good hair transplant. The proper procedures and cosmetic approaches take time and training to learn.

What the
Transplant
Cannot
Do

To avoid disappointment, the potential transplant patient must realize that although the transplanted plugs of hair will provide his naked scalp with a certain amount of natural coverage, they will not recreate the bushy mane he had at age 16. When the procedure is finished he will actually have no more hair than he had to begin with, but the hair he had will be rearranged.

The luxuriousness of hair growth in the balding areas after the procedure depends on the number of hairs contained in each plug, which ranges from six to ten hairs per 4-mm. plug. If the donor hair is sparse, the number is less. There are 100,000 hairs on the average scalp, so a vast number of plugs would be needed to cover a head that is 50 percent bald with abundant hair. One thousand plugs, said a dermatologist, would produce an excellent head of hair, but no one has enough hair in the donor sites to make 1,000 plugs. Most people need from 250 to 300 plugs to give the scalp good coverage, although the number of plugs necessary depends, of course, on the extent of hair loss. The new hair will resemble the hair on the back and sides of the head, although it might be somewhat sparser.

Patients should also realize that anyone who looks closely at their scalps will know they have had transplants because of the configuration of hair growth and the tiny circular scars surrounding each plug. Also, a less-than-lovely crust on the scalp remains for about two weeks after each transplant procedure, which some dermatologists say can be covered with a wig until new hair growth starts. Patients' transplants, in short, will be no secret from their friends.

Dermatologists say the most satisfied transplant patients are those who are mature and highly motivated, for personal or professional reasons, to obtain new hair growth. People in professional areas where a youthful image is important, politicians and people in show business, for example, are especially good candidates for the procedure. But many men find the improvement in self-image alone well worth the cost and inconvenience of the procedures. Peter M., a construction worker, said:

My hair started falling out when I was 22, right after I came home from Vietnam. I'd always had a hairline that started pretty far back on my head, and there was a lot of fuzz left, so no one really noticed it. But I panicked. I felt my whole image and personality were changing. I think most balding men feel the same—those who don't admit it, don't admit it to themselves. It affected my attitude toward girls, everything. I wouldn't go out—I just went to work and came home. The transplants improved my self-image to myself. I never much cared what other people thought of me—it wasn't that. I had seven transplant procedures and the doctor did a beautiful job. There was no pain during the procedures, and only some mild discomfort from sutures in the donor areas afterwards.

Plastic surgeons occasionally do transplants, but the procedure is almost always done by qualified dermatologists. Nonmedical, commercial salons, too, undertake the transplant procedure, but usually without proper medical supervision and often with cosmetically unsatisfactory results.

Consultation with a Physician

Although there are commercial salons and there may be doctors who will transplant the hair of anyone who walks in the office, most qualified physicians display some degree of caution as to the patients they accept. The first thing the doctor notes is the amount of hair the patient has lost and the quality of the donor site. Some patients have too small or thin a donor site, and others are not sufficiently bald to make transplant procedures worthwhile until later, when hair loss has progressed and the balding process begins to stabilize. If the patient begins having transplants the instant his hair starts to fall, he is letting himself in for an extended period of transplant procedures because every time the area behind the transplant plugs loses hair, the transplanted hair becomes an isolated island in a sea of skin. If balding is stabilized, he can have all the necessary plugs transplanted in a period of two to three months if he wishes.

Dermatologists decide the patient is ready for transplants if there is enough space between viable hair follicles to insert a 4-mm. (about ¼ inch) transplanted plug. If the patient wants to determine whether he is bald enough for transplants himself, he can draw 4-mm. circles on his head with a ruler, checking to see if there is any hair growth in a 4-mm. range. The best candidate for rejection is, therefore, the man who has just started to lose hair and has fallen into a premature state of panic. Many men want to maintain the hairline they had as children. They do not realize that hair loss is a physiological process and that the normal shape of the mature man's hairline is an M, with hair receding from the temples. Said one dermatologist:

I turned down a kid of about 19 who had a good head of hair. He said,

"It's abnormal that I should be losing hair at this age, I don't care what you say." He returned again with his father and the two of them made a terrible scene. One year later the boy was back, pretending he'd never been in my office before. After I'd rejected him he'd gone to a commercial salon and they'd given him the hairline he wanted—but it was too far forward and looked like a slightly higher version of an eyebrow. He wanted me to take the plugs out and restore his natural hairline. I don't go for telling a 19-year-old boy who comes in with most of his hair, 'My, you have a problem.' Boys should be educated to know that hair loss on the scalp is part of the physiological development of secondary sex characteristics, just like hair growth on the chin.

According to dermatologists, patients who want their restored hairline too far forward don't realize they may be creating a Count Dracula look for themselves. Untrained practitioners are apt to put the hairline wherever the patient wants it. "We see about two botched jobs a month," said one dermatologist. "They want us to take out the plugs, which we seldom do because they leave significant scars in a visible area."

Some doctors also reject patients who feel their whole lifestyle will be improved by the transplant or who imagine the procedure will endow them with the same amount of hair they had as teenagers. A good physician will try to determine the patient's motivation for the operation. If patients desiring transplants are rejected by more than one reputable physician, they should take no for an answer and not entrust their scalps to a poorly trained or nonmedical practitioner.

Preoperative
Procedure

Before the doctor begins the transplant procedure he evaluates the patient's general health, ascertains the cause of balding, and determines blood count and blood-sugar levels. Occasionally a patient evinces a blood-clotting malfunction, which would make bleeding hard to stop and prevent the transplanted plugs from taking. Black patients are also checked for deformative scarring or keloid tendencies. Patients are then given a written outline of the principles of the hair transplant operation and the procedure, advised to eat normally, but not to take alcohol for 24 hours and aspirin for seven days before the operation.

Before any hair is actually transplanted, the desired cosmetic effect and the number of procedures necessary to obtain it are discussed with the patient. The doctor may ask for pictures of the patient in his more hirsute days, and the new hairline is drawn in on the scalp.

Anesthesia

All transplant procedures are done in the doctor's office under a local anesthetic, which is injected into the scalp with a needle.

Inserting a needle into the head can be painful, so most doctors freeze the scalp first with an ethyl chloride spray, which raises a tiny, numb weal in several areas of the scalp. The air-spray injection is virtually painless itself and provides a painless entry point for the needle. Once a patient's scalp is numbed by the anesthetic, the entire procedure is almost completely painless. Confirmed one balding dermatologist:

People kept asking me, "If the transplant procedure is so terrific, why don't you have it yourself?" As a doctor I wanted to find out if there is pain during and after the operation, because I'd had some patients who complained of discomfort and others who felt none. I experienced no pain myself. Actually, I'd rather have transplants than go to the dentist any day. I suspect patients who complain of pain are nervous as cats about the procedure and are anticipating pain. Sometimes the anesthetic misses a tiny spot and they feel pain there. Usually, once the head is anesthetized you could cut it off and there'd be no pain.

The Surgical Procedure

The surgical procedure for each transplant procedure takes from one half to two hours, depending on how many plugs are done. First the doctor clips the hair in the donor sites and cleanses the area with 70 percent alcohol. Before he inserts the punch into the scalp he carefully ascertains the direction of hair growth. It is of utmost importance that he insert the punch parallel to the hair follicles, which do not send hair out of the head at right angles, but at a slant. Sometimes the hair in only one small area of the scalp may grow at different angles. If the punch is inserted at an angle different from the one in which the hair follicles lie, several of the follicles in the plug will be severed by the sharp edge of the punch and lost. The follicles rest in a bed of fat, which must also be excised to protect them. If the vacant holes in the donor site bleed heavily, the doctor sutures them; stitches are removed the following day. Later hair growth hides the small scars in the area.

The donor plugs are removed from the scalp with tweezerlike forceps and placed immediately in a dish filled with sterile saline solution. The plugs must not be allowed to dry, but can live on refrigerated in their moisturizing solution if the operation is interrupted. Then they are trimmed of excess fat and loose hair, which may cause infections. Great care is taken not to damage the base of the follicles.

As he places the plugs in their new bed, the doctor is careful to make sure that the direction of future hair growth from the plugs is in a cosmetically desirable position and in relation to whatever hair growth may already exist in the area. The hair in the hairline, for example, usually grows forward, not at right

185

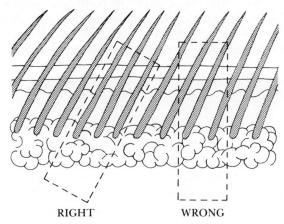

RIGHT   WRONG

When donor plugs are cut at the correct angle, the entire hair follicle is removed intact.

angles or backwards, and the hair follicles in the plugs must also point forward. Although the top of the scalp does not bleed heavily when recipient sites are prepared, the light bleeding that takes place is necessary to form clots with the transplanted plugs and connect them to the vascular supply in the new site.

The Motorized Versus the Hand Punch

Both the excision of the transplant plugs and preparation of the recipient sites are done with a small cylindrical punch, 1 to 4 mm. in diameter. Some doctors are now using a motorized version of this punch, which can perform the procedure faster and requires less hand strength and pressure on the part of the doctor.

Doctors have mixed feelings about the motorized punch. Although some claim it can zip plugs in and out faster, tiring the doctor less, others feel it does not really speed up the process since what slows the doctor down is ascertaining the right angle at which to insert the punch. Doctors also believe the motorized punch is apt to clip off hair follicles. All in all, the type of punch the doctor uses depends on his skill and familiarity with the equipment.

The Strip Technique

Sometimes physicians, particularly plastic surgeons, excise a long, narrow graft from the donor site to create a hairline. If the technique works, it forms a neater, natural looking, continuous line of hair, but there is lack of agreement on the efficacy of the technique. Dermatologists, in general, reject it because a strip is (1) a large graft which doesn't always take, and if it doesn't it can leave a sizable scar in a visible area. The rate of infection for strip grafts is higher, too; (2) the strip does not have as much flexibility as the small plugs for shaping the hairline, which normally weaves in and out; and (3) it leaves a large scar in the donor site. Said one doctor: "We're talking about a cosmetic procedure, not a life and death operation. The fewer risks, the better."

There is a difference of opinion among doctors about how many plugs should be transplanted per procedure and how many procedures are necessary. Two to five procedures are usually enough to gain the desired cosmetic effect, and they may be done in a period of two or three months. Some patients, however, prefer to stretch the procedures out to coincide with vacations, and several years may thus elapse before the procedures are completed. As already mentioned, patients who begin having transplants before the balding process has stabilized will need additional transplants when hair loss progresses further.

How Many Procedures and How Many Plugs?

In general, the first procedure serves to establish the patient's new hairline. In subsequent procedures, the areas behind the new hairline are filled. Doctors usually transplant from 10 to 60 plugs per session, although some may do as many as 100 or 200. There is danger of infection and death of the plugs if too many plugs are done at one time, and patients will be wise to avoid this. Each plug must be surrounded by normal skin, because if plugs are placed too close together they constitute, in effect, a much larger skin graft with a higher risk. Therefore, doctors don't pack a single area of the scalp with plugs, but may work on more than one area at once. In later sessions the doctor fills in spaces between previous plugs with new transplants. These new grafts can be placed in three to four weeks, and new areas can be "sodded" anytime following the previous procedure. Often smaller plugs are placed between larger plugs on the hairline to give it a more natural configuration.

After the procedure the physician anoints the patient's head with an antibiotic ointment and bandages it with a nonocclusive dressing, then with gauze—removable within 24 hours. The patient is advised not to drink alcohol for one day or in any way disturb the plugs for two weeks. A comb or brush should not be run over the graft sites. Strenuous activity should be avoided for five days. Some doctors recommend wetting the scalp after the procedure to keep the crust formation moist, but it should not be shampooed for five days. The crusts that form after the operation come off of their own accord in about 10 to 14 days. If the crust itches, the patient should avoid picking or scratching, but instead apply a soothing ointment prescribed by the doctor. If the crusts have not fallen off in two weeks, patients should not attempt to remove them. One patient said:

Postoperative Recovery Period

My head was pretty much of a mess afterwards. I couldn't wash my hair for a while and I had to keep an antibiotic gel on the bloody crusts, so my hair was all slicked down and slimy. My wife didn't seem to mind though, and never tried to deter me from having the procedures.

Doctors report that patients are anxious about the crust formation before they have the procedures, but afterwards find it to be a minimal problem. Often the crusts, which resemble the scab on a skinned knee, can be covered by combing existing hair over them.

Possible
Complications

Usually there are no medical complications following the procedure and little pain. Patients may return to work the same day. Mild discomfort, numbness of the scalp and slight bleeding, however, are not abnormal. "If a patient calls in with severe pain, I want to see him," said one dermatologist, "because it's rare. It's amazing to think we can put so many holes in a patient's head without causing him pain." If the patient experiences postoperative bleeding, he can usually stop it himself by applying local pressure to the area with a clean handkerchief. Infections at the plug sites, hematomas, merging of blood vessel walls after surgery, and keloid scarring occur, but are rare. Swelling of the forehead and eye area occur occasionally.

Most complications are cosmetic. If the doctor is not skilled and severs follicles, the plugs may not take. If the doctor does not trim plugs properly and insert them far enough into the scalp they will create a raised cobbled effect; sometimes the plugs feel raised to the touch, but do not look it. A badly designed hairline may appear peculiar, and hair from poorly positioned plugs may grow in the wrong direction. Patients should remember that hair in the plugs may fall out, but when new hairs grow they are permanent.

Fees

Dermatologists charge from $5 to $25 per plug of hair. The usual fee is $8 to $10. Costs are higher on the West Coast. Although the number of plugs a patient needs varies, depending on the extent of hair loss, the average cost of the entire cosmetic procedure is usually between $2,000 and $3,000.

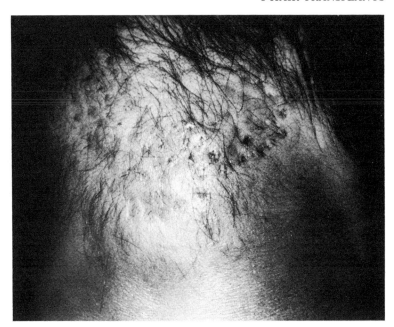

PHOTOGRAPHS COURTESY OF NORMAN ORENTREICH, M.D.

HAIR
TRANSPLANT
*Three weeks after
treatment*

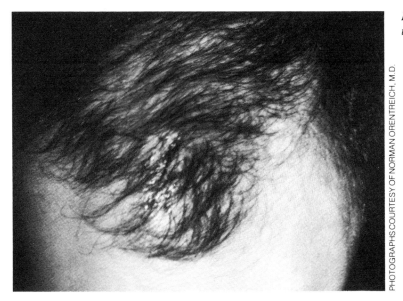

*Five months after
treatment*

9

The Breasts:

Augmentation, reduction, lifting, correction of
asymmetry, and reconstruction

The female breast, despite its enduring sexual and feminine significance and its source of nourishment for the young, has not escaped the whim and caprice of fashion. Depending on the aesthetic ideal of the period, breasts have been hidden or exposed, ballooned up by stiffened underpinnings or flattened down by shapeless bandeaus. Now the look is free and natural, the contour of the breast unmistakable and often visible under soft, clinging garments. Regardless of fashion, however, the female breast has always been an object of sensual attention for the man and a measure of womanliness and sex appeal for the woman.

Anatomically, the breasts or mammary glands are two skin-covered hemispheres filled with fatty tissue, blood and lymph vessels, nerves, and milk ducts and glands. The milk ducts open up on the nipple, which is perforated with from 15 to 20 tiny holes that fulfill the purpose for which this remarkable organ was originally designed by a provident nature. The nipple is surrounded by a halo of pigmented skin—the areola. Fatty tissue exists in considerable abundance in the breast and determines its size and form. Located on the front and sides of the chest, each breast extends from the first or second rib to the sixth or seventh rib.

A woman's breasts change at different stages of her life. At birth, breast development is about equal for both sexes. During puberty, the female breast increases rapidly to the mature state. Most of the change in size is caused by an accumulation of fat and the effect of various hormones, not all of which is completely understood. The size and shape of the breasts fluctuate, affected by menstruation, heredity, age, weight gains and losses, pregnancy, and, as with all soft tissues in the body, the relentless pull of gravity.

That not every breast develops in the same way is plainly evident in any gathering of women. To the dismay and disappointment of some women, the "budding breast" may never develop past that point, whereas in others the breasts can become so enormous that they cause not only embarrassment but

191

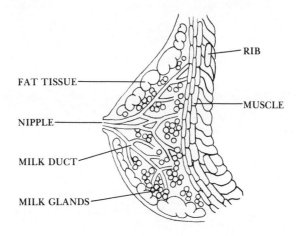

RIB

FAT TISSUE

MUSCLE

NIPPLE

MILK DUCT

MILK GLANDS

ANATOMY OF THE BREASTS

actual physical discomfort. Sometimes one breast develops normally, while the other mysteriously does not develop at all or unaccountably atrophies, resulting in marked asymmetry. A woman's breasts are rarely exact duplicates of each other. The observation that "there is no symmetry in nature" may have originated with a classical sculptor who studied many human forms during the course of his work. Nevertheless, a significant variation in size between the two breasts can be most disturbing and difficult to conceal. Then there are the drooping breasts, not overly large or small, but lacking in firmness. This condition may occur following the additional breast weight that goes along with pregnancy and lactation, and the breast may never be capable of regaining its former shape. There are some girls, however, who sag at 18 and some women who remain high and firm throughout their lives.

The correction of these defects lies within the province of the plastic surgeon. Plastic surgery of the breast—mammaplasty—can enlarge the underdeveloped breast by the insertion of a silicone implant. It can reduce the oversized pendulous breast by a major surgical procedure that involves trimming the breast tissues and the skin that covers them. Balance is brought to asymmetrical breasts either by enlarging the smaller one or reducing the larger one; in some cases it may be necessary to both reduce one breast and enlarge the other for a good result. Lifting small sagging breasts is different from enlarging them—a sagging breast cannot be corrected by an implant. The sagging breast has more skin than its volume requires, so the skin brassiere must be tightened. And there is the operation to reconstruct a breast after its removal for cancer, a procedure that is bringing great psychological benefits to many women.

Are there age limits for cosmetic surgery of the breast? Not at the far end of the age spectrum. Women in their sixties and seventies in good physical and mental health may be suitable candidates, but it is not recommended for young girls until at least two years after the onset of menstruation when the breasts reach their full development. Excellent psychological and physical improvements have resulted from the surgical correction of marked asymmetry of the breasts in 16- and 17-year-old girls, most of whom are extremely self-conscious over what they consider a deformity. To delay this surgery could mean an additional period of emotional trauma.

Ideally, aesthetic breast surgery should be undertaken when the body weight is stable, since breasts change in size in relation to weight changes. A pattern of weight loss and gain following surgery to enlarge or reduce the size of the breasts could adversely affect the result of the operation. Also, aesthetic surgery of the breast should not be performed until at least three months after a pregnancy, whether full term or interrupted. During pregnancy the breasts become engorged and there is danger of excessive bleeding unless sufficient time has elapsed for the blood to return to normal.

The obvious question that comes to the mind of those contemplating cosmetic breast surgery is the possible risk of cancer. According to informed medical opinion based on many thousands of cases, enlarging or reducing the breast does not increase the incidence of human breast cancer. It is generally accepted that about 5 to 6 percent of American women will develop breast cancer, and this percentage has not been exceeded in comprehensive studies of the group that has received implants or breast reductions.

Cosmetic surgery of the breast is not a casual undertaking and should not be considered without careful evaluation of the advantages and risks. The advantages? To give the improved body contour that will make the woman feel better and happier about herself. It is not an operation to be undertaken to please someone else or with the hope that a shapely, rounded bosom will make any appreciable difference in one's life, except for the additional self-confidence that comes with liking the way you look. The risks? As with all surgery, breast operations are not 100 percent successful and complications do occur occasionally. But there is less possibility of something going wrong when the surgeon is competent and well trained and is in good standing in an accredited hospital.

Breast augmentation or enlargement, also known as augmentation mammaplasty, is a procedure in which breasts that are too

Physical
Considerations

Breast
Augmentation

193

small, asymmetric, or atrophied are increased in size and improved in contour by the introduction into the breast of a synthetic implant. Once this procedure was considered frippery, and exclusively for women whose livelihoods depended on the proper curves being in the proper places. Today, however, 80 percent of those seeking breast augmentation are married women in their thirties with children. Breast augmentation has increased steadily in popularity since 1962 when the silicone gel implant was developed. Early in 1977 it was estimated that about three-quarters of a million women have had silicone implants in their breasts.

The Search for
Implant Material

Until the development of the silicone implant, various substances and devices were used to fill out and firm up inadequate breasts. Paraffin injections were introduced in the late 1930s with subsequent catastrophic results. In the 1940s an operation was revived that had been introduced a couple of decades earlier to reconstruct breasts removed for cancer or other diseases. Fat and fascia (fibrous tissue under the skin) were taken from the buttocks, refashioned into a conical shape, and inserted in the breasts. This left the patient with scars on the buttocks as well as on the breasts, and because fat has a tendency to be reabsorbed by the body unless an excellent blood supply is maintained, the transplants were frequently short-lived. Another method involved taking a flap of skin and fat from the abdomen and transposing it up and under the breast. This left huge scars on the abdomen. Plastic sponges of Teflon, Dacron, and Ivalon, among other products, were used for breast implants, but they all lacked the lasting qualities necessary for a successful implant.

In the 1950s, injectable liquid silicone came on the scene and was greeted with considerable enthusiasm. It seemed to be the answer to a long search for a material that would add tissue bulk to parts of the body without resorting to surgery. It has now been completely discredited. Drops of silicone in the breast tissue can mask the detection of breast cancer. Equally important, when liquid silicone is injected into the breast in large quantities, it wanders through the body, getting lost in the tissues and collecting in clumps under the skin. It is practically irretrievable. In spite of these findings, some physicians and a number of unlicensed practitioners are continuing to use silicone fluid for breast augmentation. Because medical grade liquid silicone has been made available to only eight investigators in the United States—and none for breast augmentation—the silicone used in many instances is industrial silicone which was never meant to be used in the human body. The practice cannot be condemned strongly enough. Any patient who subjects herself to injections

194

of liquid silicone for breast augmentation is accepting a most serious risk.

An implant to augment the
breast is placed against
the chest wall behind
the mammary gland.

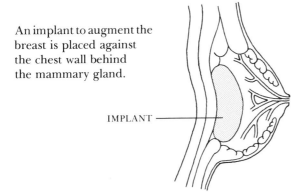

IMPLANT

Silicone implants used in breast augmentation are not to be confused with injectable liquid silicone. The most commonly used implant is either a contoured silicone envelope containing a soft silicone gel or an inflatable silicone balloon that is inserted empty into the breast, filled with a sterilized liquid, and sealed shut by closing off a valve that is then buried neatly under the balloon. The silicone implant material meets all medical criteria: it is chemically and physically stable during its contact with body tissues; it does not cause inflammation; it is nonallergenic; it can withstand stresses and strains; it can be safely sterilized, and it is noncarcinogenic. The implants are soft and resilient, and not too unlike real breasts in weight and consistency. When the implant is in position underneath the breast, the overlying breast is simple to examine and easily available for surgical biopsy should a suspicious lump appear. Silicone implants do not interfere with breast sensation, nor, it is said, with lactation, although not all plastic surgeons share this view regarding the success of nursing after augmentation surgery.

The plastic surgeon first assures himself that the patient is in satisfactory physical condition for surgery and that her reasons for wanting augmentation are sound. The woman who blames her failures in love, marriage, or career on underdeveloped breasts and expects that a larger, more feminine bosom will change her life would not be an acceptable candidate. Nor would a reluctant patient who comes to the plastic surgeon at the insistence of someone else—a mother, a husband, or a friend. Breast augmentation is an elective procedure and should be undertaken only because the patient desires it herself.

The Consultation

195

The surgeon will discuss the operative procedure with the patient and determine the size of the implant, according to his recommendations and the patient's preference. He takes into account the patient's build, size, and the amount of breast tissue present. An implant that is too large is never recommended. Not only does it increase the chance of complications, but it is less desirable aesthetically than a natural looking, unexaggerated breast.

Olga M. had a breast augmentation eight years ago. She is now in her middle forties, a tall, slim woman with the kind of figure fashion writers describe as willowy. A practicing architect, she is a member of a prestigious firm. In some ways—but not all—her breast augmentation experience was typical:

Ever since I was about 13, I've been—I can't say obsessed, that's too strong a word, maybe "bugged" would be better—about my flat chest. As a teenager I used to fantasize about a magic potion that would make my breasts sprout. I'm sure I would have sent away for most of those exotic things advertised in magazines that promise four inches in four weeks if I thought I could have gotten them past my mother. I longed for curves where my friends had them, but there I was, in padded bras and looking like a stick in a bathing suit. In any event, I grew up and married, remaining mildly neurotic about my lack of breasts.

Then one day I read an article in <u>Vogue</u> that described the augmentation operation. That was it. I made some inquiries, located a plastic surgeon and made an appointment. He agreed that I could do with a bit more bosom. It was to be made bigger, not big. The arrangements were made for the hospital, the anesthetist, and my "before" photographs. I was relieved to find that my face was not included in those photographs. In due course, the appointed day arrived.

Before
the Operation

Because of the rich blood supply in the breasts, bleeding is always a threat in breast surgery. Consequently, aspirin or any products containing it must be discontinued a full two weeks before the operation. Patients should scrupulously tell their surgeons about all medications they are taking, because some, such as those for hypertension or obesity, may be contraindicated before any surgery requiring general anesthesia and must also be discontinued well in advance.

When the operation is performed in a hospital, the patient is admitted the day before. She is instructed to bathe with an antibacterial soap and shave the areola and under the arms. Olga reminisces:

I checked into the hospital in the late afternoon. Different people wandered in and out of my room. One took blood from my arm, another a

196

urine specimen, another my blood pressure, and so on. Later in the evening the anesthetist dropped by to discuss my previous operations and to find out if I had any false teeth or allergies. Still later, the surgeon appeared. He had me stand against a hospital screen and he took more photos. With a ruler and a ball-point pen he made markings above, below, and between my breasts. It seems I was asymmetrical, as he put it, or "One Hung Low," as I put it. Bad joke.

Since I was going to have general anesthesia and not be in a position to monitor the proceedings, I was curious about the operation. The surgeon explained that an incision about 1 ½ inches is made under each breast and a pocket to house the implant is created between the chest wall and the breast. The envelope containing the silicone gel is inserted. On the back of it is a fixation patch of Dacron mesh which the fibrous tissues of the body will snake their way around, thereby securing the implant to the chest wall so it won't go flopping around. I'm told that the fixation patch isn't being used much now, but after all, this was eight years ago. Anyway, it all seemed so eminently reasonable that I took the yellow pill the nurse gave me and went to sleep without a worry.

Olga's surgeon used what is called an inframammary approach for the implantation, with the incision made under the breast fold. This is probably the most commonly used technique, one which some surgeons consider the quickest and most reliable. In what is called the areolar approach, an incision is made around the outside border of the lower half of the areola—from 3 o'clock to 9 o'clock is how the surgeons pinpoint its position. The proponents of the areolar approach favor it because, although it is more difficult to insert the implant through the limited opening, it leaves the most inconspicuous scars. Still another approach is one in which the implant is introduced into the breast through an incision in the armpit. This leaves no scar on the breast, and the one in the armpit is hidden from view. There is a considerable distance to be channeled from the armpit to the breast, but the surgeons who use this approach are most enthusiastic about it.

The most widely used implant is a soft silicone gel enclosed within a contoured silicone envelope. It comes in a wide variety of sizes and shapes. The surgeon must use his discretion in choosing the best size and shape for each patient. Some surgeons use it with the Dacron fixation patch, others prefer it without. Still others favor the silicone balloons filled with saline solution. These balloons have certain advantages, particularly for asymmetric breasts, since the bags are inserted empty and can be filled with more or less liquid to make the two breasts match in size. The bags also require a smaller incision. The antiballoon doctors point out the risks of leaks and ruptures occurring in the

The Operation for Implantation

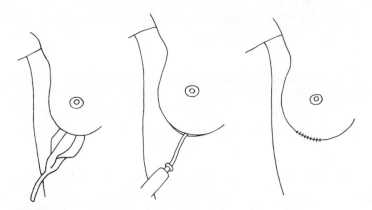

For breast augmentation, a small incision is made and an empty
silicone balloon is inserted. (Some surgeons insert the balloon through
an incision along the areola). Saline solution is injected into the
balloon through a tube. The tube is then trimmed and sealed,
and the incision is closed.

balloons, an allegation disputed by their champions, who claim
that the bags have been improved and the danger of leaks is
slight.

Breast augmentation may be done under local or general
anesthesia, according to the choice of the surgeon and patient.
General anesthesia is always used for patients who are apprehensive and fearful of being conscious during surgery. Local
anesthesia is combined with sedation and epinephrine (Adrenalin) to reduce bleeding during surgery.

After the skin of the chest from above the collar bone to the
end of the rib cage is thoroughly scrubbed and disinfected, the
surgeon makes the incision according to the markings he drew
on the patient's chest while she was sitting upright. He prepares
a pocket behind each mammary gland, where it contacts the
chest muscles. All blood vessels that are exposed are meticu-
lously closed off with electrocautery to avoid hematomas
(swellings caused by a collection of blood). The pockets are irri-
gated with saline solution to wash out loose fat particles and
blood clots. When the areas are completely free of bleeding, the
surgeon carefully inserts the implants, making sure they are
symmetrical and in exactly the right position. The incisions are
closed and the wounds are dressed according to the choice of the
surgeon. Often the patient is put into a snug-fitting bra.

When this operation is done as an outpatient procedure, the
patient rests for a short period and returns home with medication for pain and sleeping.

Patients are not restricted in their activities as they once were. In the past, patients were told that they *must* sleep on their backs, that they must *not* raise their arms above their heads for a month or lift anything, but the majority of surgeons are now much more relaxed about rules. The patient may find she is more comfortable when she sleeps on her back, but it is not mandatory that she do so. Patients should postpone vigorous activities such as playing tennis or swimming for three to four weeks, but other than that they may do anything they are comfortable with—within reason.

Postoperative management after breast augmentation varies with each surgeon. Some surgeons give a massive injection of an antibiotic immediately following surgery. Others may prescribe antibiotics by mouth for a number of days following surgery, and some omit antibiotics entirely. Some surgeons change dressings after 48 hours and others do not disturb them for a week. The schedule for the removal of stitches also varies. But all patients are advised to wear a stretch bra continuously for a number of months and are advised against ever wearing brassieres that have stays or bones.

Did Olga have any great discomfort after the operation for breast augmentation?

I never had any real pain. I felt achy and stuffy the first day or two after the operation. . . . My main complaint was a backache. The doctor said it might have been a muscle cramp from lying on my back since I couldn't turn on my side, but it finally went away and by the time I left the hospital three days after the operation, I was fine.

A week after the operation, I had my unveiling. I had gone to the doctor earlier that day looking rather odd with my squarish bosom created by the wad of foam rubber I was wrapped in. What a relief when he took it off! I managed to get a look at the new bosom which was a peculiar yellow because of whatever it was that was painted on before the operation. The doctor removed some of the stitches—he said he was leaving half of them in, but I couldn't see what he was doing over my new shelf. I didn't believe it was all me and I couldn't really feel that it was.

Anyway, I had to wait until I got home to see what was really going on, and then I put off looking for a while. Then, finally, I examined myself critically in the mirror. Not bad. I thought I looked . . . well, normal . . . like everybody else. My bosom was neither large nor small . . . just right, I thought.

As in all surgery, unforeseen complications can occur during and after the operation. Infection, though infrequent, does occur. It is treated by the proper use of antibiotics and drainage. In some cases, the removal of the implant may be indicated.

Complications

199

Hematoma is always a danger and every effort is made during surgery to avoid this by scrupulously cauterizing or ligating all bleeding points during surgery. Hematomas that cannot be reabsorbed must be surgically treated. Prompt attention to this complication will usually prevent loss of the implant.

Sometimes healing of the wound is interrupted. There are many causes, ranging from infection to fluid accumulation, hematoma, improper support, or pressure against the wound from a wired brassiere or from trauma. Occasionally, the outline of the implant can be seen or felt in women who have very little fat on the chest wall and the uppermost part of the breast. In some cases the pressure of the implant can cause breakdown of the skin and it should be brought to the attention of the surgeon and watched.

A fairly common and unwelcome sequel to breast augmentation is undesirable firmness of the breasts. This comes about because of the body's natural process of surrounding any foreign object placed within it with fibrous tissue. In some women—and no one understands exactly why—the tissues surrounding the implant form into a membrane that contracts, and instead of the implant lying soft and squashed against the chest, it is squeezed into a hard ball. This contracture may begin anywhere from 2 to 12 weeks after implantation. Some surgeons believe that at least 30 percent of women having breast augmentation develop the contracture.

Hard, shrunken implants can be both painful and embarrassing for the patient. As treatment, some surgeons recommend the squeeze-and-break method— breaking the capsule by applying a great deal of pressure around the periphery of the breasts. It is successful in some cases, but too often the firmness recurs. The other method of dealing with this condition is to remove the implant along with the fibrous capsule and to replace it with a smaller implant of a different type, with the hope that it will not happen again. There is no way of anticipating the outcome. Plastic surgeons hope one day to find a sure way to avoid this untoward result. Olga hopes so, too.

It dawned on me a few years ago that my breasts were extraordinarily hard —so hard, in fact, that I couldn't sleep on my stomach. I didn't go back to see the doctor because of the everlasting wait in his office. I just didn't have the time. Incidentally, why don't doctors pay more attention to the way their secretaries book appointments? No one expects to be taken exactly on the minute of an appointment, but a wait of hours and hours is unconscionable. Anyway, I was annoyed with the doctor about that, and when the breasts began to harden, it ticked me off further. Of course, now I understand that this capsuling was not his fault, although in the beginning I did blame him. I can't say I'm happy with the result. . . . For one thing, the nipples are too low. My bosom looks like Snoopy's nose in profile . . . but in spite of all this, I would rather have had the operation than not. I certainly look better in sweaters and bathing suits than before. And I'm not giving up—yet. I have an appointment next week with another plastic surgeon and I'll see what he suggests.

Fees for breast augmentation range from $1,000 to $2,500. **Fees** Some surgeons bill the silicone implants separately and others include them in the fee. The silicone gel prostheses range from $175 to $225 a pair. When general anesthesia is used, the anesthesiologist's fee ranges from $200 to 20 percent of the surgeon's fee. Since breast augmentation is an elective, aesthetic operation, it is not covered by insurance plans.

Most women interested in breast augmentation are concerned **Breast Reduction** with achieving a more feminine contour. Breast reduction (reduction mammaplasty), in contrast, is generally sought for reasons other than a preoccupation with the aesthetic advantages of gravity-defying breasts. Reduction mammaplasty may be considered a cosmetic procedure, but it is often prompted by physical necessity. Massive, pendulous breasts (a condition called macromastia or hypertrophy) can, by their weight, provoke severe backache and neck pains, postural defects, and furrowed shoulders from brassiere straps. Often the skin under the breasts is chronically irritated. Young girls particularly suffer mental agonies with this condition. What appears voluptuous to others seems grotesque to them. It doesn't matter that their girl friends are envious and boys ogle them.

Many different techniques have been described for reducing breasts since interest in the operation arose in the early 1920s. Scores of surgeons from Europe and from North and South America have developed various methods, all with the same aim of creating normal-looking, symmetrical breasts with sensitive, erectile nipples. Scars remain after breast reduction that are permanent and visible but the women who have exchanged them for the physical and psychological comfort of more average-sized breasts consider it a highly worthwhile trade.

The two principal methods of reducing breast size are the reduction mammaplasty in which the nipple is separated from the gland and replaced, and the reduction mammaplasty in which the nipple is transposed. The latter does not touch the muscles, nerves, or superficial blood vessels and preserves the nursing function of the breast, but transplantation is sometimes necessary when the breasts are very large. The surgeon has

201

sound medical reasons for his choice of method, based on the best interests of the patient. Neither technique should affect the normal reaction of the nipple to stimulus.

Patient Selection

Reduction mammaplasty is major surgery. The general physical condition of the patient is important because she will be immobilized on the operating table under general anesthesia between two and four hours. Patients with lung disease tolerate anesthesia poorly, and healing may be delayed in those with arteriosclerosis or other circulatory diseases. Diabetes and marked obesity also increase risks. There is always the possibility of complications when massive amounts of tissue are removed. Pregnancy is a firm contraindication to breast surgery.

There are many borderline cases where judgment must prevail over symptoms. For example, a woman with massive breasts and moderate cardiopulmonary disease may be helped by breast reduction, which lessens the strain on her heart and eases the mechanical act of breathing.

The Operation for Breast Reduction

No single account can reflect all of the techniques used by plastic surgeons to reduce breasts. The basic steps entail removal of excess skin and breast tissue, reshaping the remaining breast, and repositioning the nipple.

Before the patient is anesthetized in the operating room, the surgeon marks on her chest the incision lines he will follow. Some surgeons prefer that the patient be in a sitting position for preoperative measurements and markings. The surgeon indicates in colored ink the future position of the nipples and the

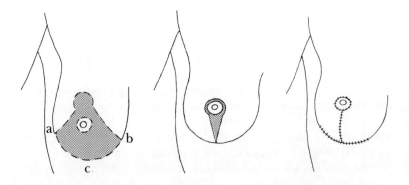

For breast reduction, excess skin and tissue are excised according to premarked guidelines. Shaping of the breast is started by suturing the lower corners of the skin flaps, a and b, to the mark on the submammary fold, c. The areola is then sutured in place and all wounds are closed.

submammary fold (fold under the breast). Some surgeons use a breast pattern called a template in the preoperative markings, which is helpful in obtaining symmetry of the breasts.

The patient is then anesthetized and the surgeon proceeds with the operation, excising portions of the breast tissue and skin according to the premarked guidelines. A circular portion of the skin is excised to make space for the areola, which is lifted and fitted into place. The wounds are then closed. The final steps are the suturing of the vertical incision from the nipple to the breast fold underneath, and the horizontal incision along the breast fold. This particular technique results in an inverted T-shaped scar.

Some surgeons insert a small drainage tube through the lower incision to prevent accumulation of fluids. Dressings vary with the choice of the surgeon.

After the Operation

The patient may or may not be confined to bed for the first day or two following surgery, depending on the wishes of her doctor. The usual hospital stay is anywhere from three to five days. Antibiotics are prescribed at the discretion of the surgeon. Timetables for the removal of bandages and sutures vary. Generally sutures are removed, a portion at a time, between the fourth and twenty-first days postoperatively. Patients are advised to wear a well-fitted brassiere continuously for at least a month. In most women, the scars on the breast will gradually fade and become less noticeable.

Most surgeons do not restrict their patients' arm movements, as was formerly done. Here again, judgment and common sense should prevail. The patient should not swim or play tennis for three to four weeks, but except for such vigorous activities, she may do anything she is comfortable with that does not impose a strain on her. For the first few weeks, the patient is seen by the surgeon at weekly intervals for postoperative follow-up and stitch removal, with subsequent visits spaced further apart.

Complications

Complications of varying degrees of severity may occur after reduction mammaplasty. The minor problems range from temporary disturbance of circulation in the nipple, areola, or skin flaps to stitch abscesses and slight localized wound separation. Massive wound infections are rare, particularly when proper antiseptic skin preparation before surgery has been observed.

A major complication, although a rare one, is partial or total loss of the nipple or areola. In such instances, a new areola and nipple are reconstructed with tissue from the genital region. Another negative result is a marked variation in size and shape between the two breasts. Perfect symmetry is difficult to achieve and a certain degree of asymmetry must be expected. Asymmetry or malpositioning of areola and nipple is also fairly common after mammaplasty. After surgery, nipples have a tendency to ride upward as the breasts sag from gravity. This is why many surgeons recommend that the nipples be located slightly lower than seems appropriate at the time of the operation.

Excessive scarring along the horizontal incisions underneath the breasts occasionally occurs. In some cases they are hypertrophic and in others'true keloids. Scarring may be treated by cortisone injections or surgical scar revisions followed by x-ray.

Rarely are nipple sensation and erectility completely or permanently lost after breast reduction, although it may take a number of months before the functions return.

Fees

Reduction mammaplasty fees range from $2,500 to $5,000. Since it is a lengthy operation with a longer hospital stay, both anesthesiologist's fee and hospital costs will be higher than for breast augmentation. In some situations, where the breasts are symptomatic, the breast reduction operation may be partially reimbursed by insurance.

A Patient's Experience

Joanne H. is 29 years old and the mother of a 17-month-old daughter. Joanne is 5 feet tall and her 90 pounds are perfectly distributed over a tiny, graceful, full-bosomed body. She has a dancer's body, which is not strange, since Joanne is a dancer.

I always had a firm, full bosom —a family characteristic —but when I was 22, my breasts suddenly began to enlarge. It was wild. In one year, I went from a 32C to a 36D brassiere, with no gain in weight. The doctors couldn't account for it. Hormonal imbalance was as close as anyone came to a diagnosis. My breasts became great pendulous appendages that hung to my waist. They were so heavy and painful that I had to wear a bra constantly, even when I went to bed or took a shower. My back and shoulders ached constantly from the weight.

Joanne realized that the dance career she had always hoped for had become an impossible dream, so off she went to law school away from home. She found herself thinking more and more about breast surgery, almost to the point of obsession. By the time she graduated from law school three years later, she had made up her mind about her future. It was dancing she wanted and not law, but first there was this bizarre body to take care of.

I was frightened of the operation and I guess I was afraid of being criticized for being self-indulgent and egocentric. My mother and sister gave me a lot of encouragement and support ... they understood the

204

situation because they had seen me undressed. On the other hand, my father—who didn't know what we knew—said absolutely not. No operation. Ridiculous, he said. I must explain that once those huge appendages were tucked into the specially constructed brassieres I wore, the effect was not too grotesque, I suppose. Just enough to elicit wolf whistles and comments from construction gangs and passing truck drivers. How I hated that! But then our family doctor prevailed on my father to change his mind.

Joanne's first visit with the plastic surgeon discouraged her. He agreed about the necessity for the operation and explained each step of the surgical procedure. Joanne had thought that it would be a simple operation, but when she heard that the nipple would have to be excised and repositioned and that she could never nurse a child, she had second thoughts. A psychiatrist she had been seeing for a problem unrelated to her physical condition was no help. He assured her that her wish for the operation was based on a deep-seated desire for self-mutilation. He later tried to make amends, but needless to say, he lost a patient.

I was torn with fears and conflicts. And then I thought, if my breasts hung down to my waist when I was 25, what would they be like when I was 35 or 40? A few weeks later, I was in the hospital. Only my fiancé and family knew the real reason. . . . We told friends that I was having some benign cysts removed. In retrospect, I think that was silly. Why should I have been so self-conscious about it? Now I feel no hesitancy in discussing the operation.

The operation and the postoperative period were uneventful. Joanne was kept in bed heavily sedated for two days after surgery. She does not recall any pain in the region of the incisions but she did suffer from extremely severe back pains. Her chest was covered with large bandages over cotton-wool padding. She was discharged from the hospital after a week. Because of the restrictions about raising her arms, she needed help each day with dressing and combing her hair. Joanne recalls her dismay when she first saw her breasts after the dressings were removed.

Not pretty. There were hundreds of tiny black stitches around the areola and under the breasts, which were incredibly discolored. I couldn't imagine that they would ever be smooth and firm and normal looking. But it happened! And the results were worth every moment of the pain and discomfort that went before. You can't imagine the joy of being able to dress like other people—in halters and bikinis and plain old T-shirts. A few months later, I was performing with a dance group.

Six months after the operation, Joanne was married, and a child was born two and a half years later. During pregnancy, the breasts reacted normally, increasing in size and with the usual amount of discomfort and feeling of fullness. In spite of these symptoms, Joanne realized she would not be able to nurse the baby. Today the hairline scars around the areola and on and under the breasts are scarcely visible. She has full sensation in the breasts, and the nipples become erect. She wears a brassiere to discourage sagging, although even after having had a child her breasts are firm enough not to need one.

I did make one mistake though. The surgeon had suggested that, in view of my size, my breasts be reduced to an A cup or B cup size. But since I come from a large-breasted family, I'd always seen myself as well-rounded, and I insisted on the C cup. I'm still wearing that size, but since the baby was born, I fill it out a bit more. I should have taken the doctor's advice and settled for a smaller size.

Breast Lifting

Drooping (ptosis) of the breasts, can occur in any size breast, even the very smallest. Pregnancies, weight loss, or premature aging, all aided by the relentless pull of gravity, conspire to rob the breast of its youthful contour. It sags. The nipples no longer look heavenward. There is too much skin for the content of the breast. A sagging breast, however small, is not corrected by increasing its size with implants—the patient will only end up with breasts fuller than before, still drooping. Aesthetic improvement can be achieved only by an operation that elevates the nipple to its proper site and tightens the skin brassiere.

As in a face lift, the excess skin is removed and a new contour emerges. This operation is called a skin (or dermal) mastopexy. In spite of its somewhat formidable sound, mastopexy simply means surgical fixation of a pendulous breast. It is the operation of choice when there is adequate breast volume, or as a first step in combination with augmentation when the breast volume is insufficient and a larger breast is desired. It is also a recommended procedure for a flat, pendulous breast, which may be augmented at the same time or at a later procedure.

A skin mastopexy is not designed or intended as an alternative for a breast reduction. Large breasts that droop require a reduction in size and weight and the skin mastopexy does not attempt more than minor adjustments in breast volume.

The scars that result will be the same as those from a breast reduction since the areola and nipple must be transposed and excess skin removed. There will be a vertical scar on the lower half of the breast itself in addition to the one under the breast that is concealed in the breast fold. In a person who heals well, these scars generally fade and become inconspicuous.

The surgical procedure is similar to that for reduction mammaplasty, except that little of the breast tissue is disturbed. If the breast is going to be augmented, it can be done at the time of the skin mastopexy by making the conventional pocket in back of the breast through the submammary fold region and inserting the implant before the submammary incision is closed. The operation is done under general anesthesia.

Postoperative care and restrictions are the same as those following breast reduction. Some surgeons recommend that a supportive bra be worn day and night for four to six months after a skin mastopexy, and as often as possible after that.

Some plastic surgeons suspect that with the ever-increasing popularity of breast augmentation using foreign transplants, there will be a corresponding increase in drooping of augmented breasts, and consequently an increase in the need for skin mastopexies. Since this operation affects only superficial tissues, it is possible to repeat it as often as necessary.

Fees

Fees range from $1,500 to $3,000 and upward without augmentation. Augmentation entails an additional fee of about $1,000.

Correction of Asymmetrical Breasts

Most women's breasts are not exactly symmetrical and a slight difference in size and shape is not generally a matter of concern. However, there are instances when the disparity between breasts is so marked that it creates what amounts to a deformity that can trigger a psychological problem. No one understands why one breast develops normally and the other remains abnormally small or grows to huge proportions. In either situation, asymmetry can create all sorts of emotional conflicts with a distortion of self-image that can be most damaging to a young woman. Even clothing becomes a problem—the fitting of brassieres, bathing suits, and other garments can be difficult and costly.

Most patients who come to the plastic surgeon with this problem are in their teens to early-to-midtwenties. Plastic surgeons who have studied a sizable number of patients with marked asymmetry have found that the majority of them are unusually shy, withdrawn, and embarrassed during consultation and examination. Their psychological improvement and personality change after surgery were marked. In a number of cases where the patients were overweight—probably related to their unhappiness—the improvement in their appearance resulted in their losing weight and taking renewed interest in their grooming.

Corrective Procedures

The goals in the surgical treatment of asymmetry of the breast are breasts that are similar in size and shape, a pleasing appearance, and a contour in harmony and balance with the body. However, these ideals cannot always be achieved. Perfection may not be possible, but improvement can usually be effected.

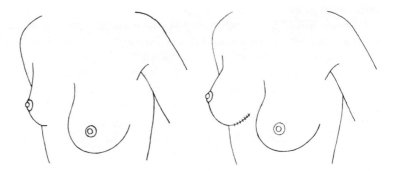

For severe asymmetry of the breasts, the underdeveloped breast is enlarged with an implant.

The overdeveloped breast then is reduced to match it. When the asymmetry is slight, only one of these operations may be needed.

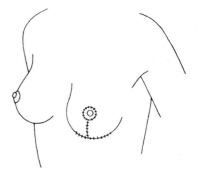

Surgical techniques to create proper balance of the breasts depend on the type of pathology present. When one breast is incompletely developed and the other is normal size, the underdeveloped breast is augmented with a silicone implant to match the normal one. However, if the normal breast droops, it will have to be corrected to match the augmented breast. In some situations, the patient may wish the larger breast to be reduced to the size of the smaller one.

If both breasts are incompletely developed but are unequal in size, augmentation with different-sized implants is indicated. In some cases, size can be controlled more precisely by using inflatable implants. The surgeon is then faced with the additional challenge of seeing to it that the nipples are level with each other. It may be necessary to reposition the lower nipple to the level of the upper.

When one breast is overly developed (hypertrophic) and the other normal, and one or both droop, the amount of reduction of the larger breast will be determined by the size of the smaller. Matching the two breasts is more difficult than the reduction of two hypertrophic breasts.

When one breast is underdeveloped and the other hypertrophic, simultaneous augmentation and reduction are indicated. The augmentation is generally done first and the reduction follows to match the size of the augmented breast as closely as possible.

The surgeon's fee, choice of anesthesia, postoperative care, convalescence, and so on, are determined by the extent of the procedures necessary.

Fees

Occasionally excessive development of the breasts occurs in normal men. Called gynecomastia, it is caused by an endocrine imbalance. Generally it has no clinical significance, but it can be a source of great embarrassment. It may have its onset at puberty and persist through adolescence. The breast enlargement may subside spontaneously but if it presents a serious psychological problem, surgical removal of the breasts may be indicated. Gynecomastia can also appear in later life. It should not be confused with pseudogynecomastia, which is an enlargement of the male breast due to deposits of fat.

Male Breast Reduction

The surgery to correct enlarged male breasts generally entails a hospital procedure with the patient under either general or local anesthesia. An incision is usually made around the lower half of the areola. It is less commonly done by an incision in the breast fold underneath the breast, since this will leave a visible scar. Glandular tissue, fat, and occasionally excess skin are removed and the incision is closed. The nipple is not disturbed. The wound is dressed according to the choice of the surgeon. The patient is discharged the day following the operation. Stitches are removed within a week.

The Operation for Enlarged Male Breasts

Fees range from $1,000 to $2,000. The operation may be covered by insurance.

Fees

Most women during the aftermath of a mastectomy (removal of a breast) go through a period of emotional peaks and valleys that ranges from joyful relief to anger and despair. The patient tries to quiet her fears by reminding herself that the unhealthy growth has been removed; she has survived a rugged bout with surgery and as a result she has earned a renewed hold on life. In

Breast Reconstruction

the hospital, she is bolstered by the reassurances of her doctor and the attention of family and friends. But the initial reactions of relief and thankfulness dim after a while—it is difficult to sustain indefinitely a feeling of being grateful—and once the patient has resumed her normal activities, she may begin to feel that she has paid for the gift of life by the loss of a vital part of her body, a part that symbolized her femininity.

Not all women react this way. Some are able to gather their courage, make peace with their disfigurement, and go on with the help of a padded bra as if there had been no mastectomy. For others, breast amputation inflicts a psychic trauma that distorts the woman's idea of herself and her feeling about how others, particularly sexual partners, regard her. Justified or not, these negative feelings are real to her, and negative feelings often defy truth and logic.

The general surgeon who performs the mastectomy has just one goal. It is to save the patient's life by removing the malignant growth and all the tissues directly or indirectly affected by it. This may necessitate a radical mastectomy, which means removing the breast, the chest muscle, and the lymph glands near the armpit and as far away as the shoulder. The modified radical procedure leaves the chest muscle, removing only the breast and the lymph glands; a simple mastectomy means breast removal only. Whichever operation is required, the melancholy result is an unfamiliar, flat, scarred chest surface. General surgeons equate their success with cure; they are less concerned with the cosmetic aspects.

Barbara A. is one of the thousands of women who discovered, quite accidentally, the tiny lump in the breast that became the prelude to a period of intense anxiety that culminated in the sound of the dreaded word—cancer. Barbara is a petite, slim, vivacious woman, looking absurdly young to be the mother of three children, ranging from 7 to 17. She remembers vividly the day, two and a half years earlier, when the surgeon telephoned her with the dire news of the laboratory report on the fluid he had removed from her breast:

I was determined at that moment to make the best of it and not punish my husband and children with this horrid thing that had happened to me. I didn't want any sympathy. All I wanted was to get in and out of the hospital as quickly as possible. And I did. I was in the hospital two days later, home a week after the operation, and by the end of the next week, I was back at my usual routine. I used my arm so much, in fact, that I scarcely needed to do the prescribed exercises.

I tried not to dwell on what had happened. I wore very expensive and very uncomfortable brassieres with a falsie, which periodically I would forget to put into the bra. One of life's embarrassing moments. All my clothes had high necks; bathing suits were specially made and equipped. I did all the usual things women have to do in this situation. The operation was a modified radical and the surgeon was most pleased with the results. Of course my husband and I were grateful that everything went well and that I was alive and had every prospect for continuing. But that didn't stop me from rebelling inwardly and feeling, well, mutilated is the only word I can think of.

About a year after the operation a friend told me about a magazine article she had read that described breast reconstruction after a mastectomy and then, a day or two later, there was a story in our local newspaper about the same operation being performed by one of the plastic surgeons in our town. I had never heard of the operation before and my surgeon had never mentioned that such a procedure was possible. I telephoned the plastic surgeon that very same day for an appointment.

Plastic surgery for breast reconstruction after mastectomy is not new; it has been done for the past 50 years. However, it is only within the last decade or so that improved breast implants together with refinements of surgical techniques have produced more aesthetically successful results. Some general surgeons are reluctant to give their patients information about breast reconstruction, perhaps out of fear of raising false hopes, or perhaps because of conservatism and the feeling that the patient should learn to accept her situation.

Not every patient is suitable for breast reconstruction. When radical mastectomy has previously made skin grafting necessary or has left scar tissue surrounded by tight, delicate skin, or when extensive radiation has damaged the tissues, the painful, time-consuming procedures necessary to graft skin from other parts of the body—thereby creating more scars—may not justify the aesthetic results of the breast restoration. In cases where the incision has healed well and there is sufficient skin and no evidence of inflammation or recurrence, the plastic surgeon may be able to do a great deal to restore a woman's self-image. The restoration is usually performed 6 to 12 months after the mastectomy—sometimes sooner, but rarely at the same time.

Barbara talks of her meeting with the plastic surgeon:

I floated into his office, brimming with expectations, and I left shattered. The doctor explained what could be done and he showed me the silicone gel implant that he uses. He was very blunt about the final result. He made it clear that the breast would not look perfect. He said he could give me a contour but he couldn't restore a breast that looked exactly like my own. He thought I had enough skin on my chest to accommodate an A cup brassiere, but since I had always worn a C cup, the other breast

211

would have to be reduced for the sake of symmetry. Of course he could see how upset I was and he suggested that I think about it for the next few weeks and make my decision. It was the first time since this whole thing started that I cried. I cried all the way home from his office.

The objective in breast reconstruction is to restore the normal breast contour when the patient is wearing a brassiere. In some cases, the reconstructed breast may look nearly normal, but this is the exception rather than the rule. The really striking visible improvement—aside from the psychological one—is in the restoration of the natural cleavage between the breasts, which can never be simulated by a padded bra. The patient can wear low-cut clothes with complete ease.

The patient must also understand that there is still no effective treatment for the hollow resulting after a radical mastectomy that is produced by the loss of the uppermost part of the main chest muscle, although attempts have been made to replace it with a silicone prosthesis. However, some cancer surgeons, with an eye to future reconstruction, are now endeavoring to leave this part of the muscle intact, which allows great improvement in the postoperative appearance. They are also trying, when performing the mastectomy, to use a horizontal incision instead of the classic vertical one, thereby making the restoration easier.

The type of implant that is used in breast reconstruction depends on the personal preference of the plastic surgeon. Some use the standard Cronin silicone gel implant popularly used in breast augmentation, while others prefer the Ashley type, which is a silicone envelope covered with polyurethane. It is constructed in such a way that it maintains the breast shape. The champions of this implant maintain that the design and covering of it give the result a more "natural feel." There is also a made-to-measure prosthesis that duplicates the size and shape of the natural breast.

The surgeon does not try to match the natural breast perfectly. The implant must be small because an overly large one will produce tension in the skin that could induce rejection. He may use a small inflatable bag first, and when the skin has stretched, insert a larger implant. Or the decision may be made to reduce the natural breast.

The Operation   For the next few days Barbara was filled with doubt and uncertainty. Should she subject herself to more surgery only to face disappointment? Was it worth the risk? She spoke to the surgeon who operated on her originally. He strongly opposed the reconstruction operation. He said it was unnecessary and unsafe, and chided her for not contenting herself with the fact that her life had been saved. "If it were my wife, I wouldn't permit it," he told her.

Finally Barbara made up her mind. She was 39 years old, which, according to actuarial tables plus a bit of luck, gave her the prospect of almost as many years ahead as there were behind her. To achieve even a degree of normalcy was a chance worth taking. She asked the plastic surgeon to send the cancer surgeon an account of the operation being planned. In due course the reply came, giving approval.

Once again, Barbara packed her suitcase, but this time for a three-day hospital stay, and with a feeling of happy anticipation understandably missing on her previous hospital visit.

The surgeon had assured me that this operation would be less painful than the former one. Since there was practically no pain to speak of with that operation—physical pain, that is, the emotional trauma was something else—I wasn't anticipating any problems. But after I regained consciousness I was in the throes of the most hideous pain I have ever experienced. I felt as if my chest were being torn apart. I wished that the surgeon had warned me that this might happen so that I could have been better prepared for it. I've been told since that this is most unusual so I suppose the surgeon had no way of knowing it would occur. It lasted for two more days and gradually diminished. For the first 24 hours I had to be flat on my back to give the breast time to settle into its new home. I recall how heavy it felt for the first few days. After all, for a long time there had been nothing there, but I soon got used to it.

There were some pleasant surprises. The surgeon had told me that he would delay placing the nipple on the new breast but during the operation he changed his mind. He used some of the nipple tissue which he took from the other breast when he reduced it. The nipple is a bit off center but that doesn't bother me in the least. And then he found there was more skin to work with than he had anticipated, so instead of an A cup, he was able to give me a B cup. I returned home the day after the operation and had an uneventful convalescence.

The breast reconstruction operation is usually performed under general anesthesia although some surgeons do it under local. The approximate position for the new breast is marked off before the operation. The surgeon makes an incision on the chest and dissects a pocket for the implant. The method of insertion is much the same as that used in breast augmentation. The implant is positioned and the wound is closed in layers. Sometimes drainage tubes are inserted. Dressings vary with the choice of the surgeon. Some surgeons tape a small dressing over the suture line but nothing over the reconstructed breast. This is to prevent pressure on the skin flap and to allow frequent observation of the breast for the first 24 hours. The result at this point is a properly positioned, adequately sized mound. The shape will gradually improve during the first year as the skin stretches.

Although Barbara's surgeon reconstructed a nipple simultaneously with the operation, many surgeons prefer to postpone this step for about three months. There are a number of methods for reconstruction of the areola. The original areola can be stored as a graft after the mastectomy by being implanted immediately on the patient's leg or abdomen. Some doctors consider that the use of the original areola risks spread of the malignancy, but others feel that in cases where the tumor in the breast was small and a good distance away from the nipple, it is safe to use it after it has been properly biopsied and found negative for cancer cells. An areola may be tattooed, or, as in Barbara's case, the surgeon can use tissue from the other breast's nipple. Nipple skin may also be taken from the genital region because it is the best part of the body in which to find the correct color. This last is the choice of many doctors; the procedure is relatively painless and minor and gives excellent cosmetic results. Restoring the nipple is a simple and quick operation, but many patients are content with the improvement in contour and do not bother to return to have the nipple rebuilt. The operation for a breast restoration takes about an hour and has a postoperative course requiring practically no care. What are the rewards? Barbara talks about them:

This last year and a half, since my breast reconstruction, has been a new life for both my husband and me. I feel whole again. Most of the time I don't remember which breast is the real one. I get up in the morning and dress without thinking about camouflage and covering up. Everything is better—golf, tennis, sex, dancing. I would never say this before, but after the mastectomy I felt like a freak, and I don't feel like a freak anymore. I can change my clothes in the locker room at the club without cringing if someone comes in. I find myself buying clothes I wouldn't have dreamed of even five years ago. Why, the other night I wore a halter-neck dress cut way down. A shocking dress, really. No brassiere and perfect cleavage. Would you believe it?

The question that naturally comes up is whether the breast reconstruction can trigger a recurrence of the malignancy. Informed medical opinion agrees that there is no evidence at this time to suggest that an implant can revive a cancerous tumor that has been completely removed. However, in cancer-prone women, or in women with a strong family history of cancer, there is always the possibility that certain forms of malignancy may appear in the second breast. To avoid this, some surgeons recommend a double mastectomy. This may appear a heroic procedure, but it removes the threat of future malignancies and some specialists in this field advocate it under certain conditions.

An operation called a subcutaneous mastectomy is sometimes performed on the healthy breast. This involves removal of the glandular breast tissue, leaving intact the overlying skin and nipple. It may be followed immediately by an implant to restore the shape of the breast. Not all surgeons are in agreement about the effectiveness of this procedure; some feel that it is inadequate in a cancer-prone breast since the remaining breast tissue and areola and nipple may harbor some cancer cells.

Infection and hematomas (swelling caused by a collection of blood) are rare after breast reconstruction. The too-early reconstruction of the areola can result in a fistula of the areola. Occasionally there is impairment of the circulation of the skin covering the implant. Removal of the implant with later reinsertion of the same size implant is generally successful.

Complications

Fees for breast reconstruction range from $1,500 to $5,000, depending on the surgeon, the geographical area, and the extent of the surgery. In some states, Blue Cross and Blue Shield will pay hospital costs and part of the surgical fees for breast reconstruction after mastectomy.

Fees

BREAST RECON-
STRUCTION
AFTER
MASTECTOMY
Before

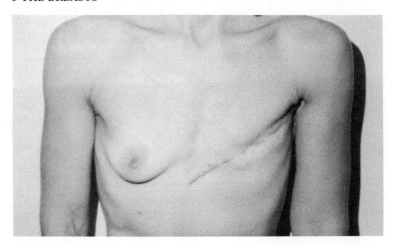

After

Augmentation of right breast; reconstruction of left breast

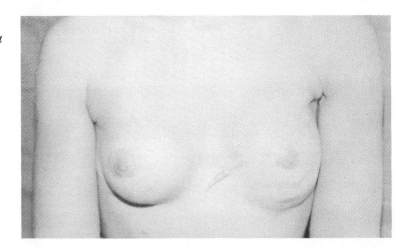

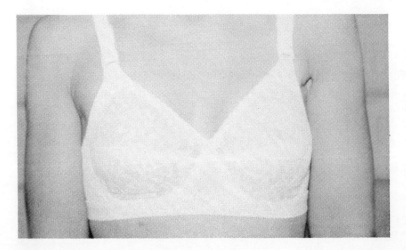

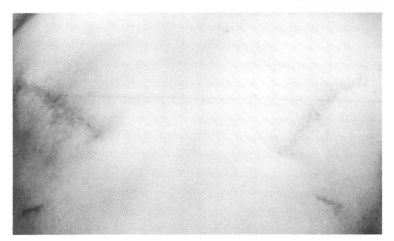

DOUBLE
MASTECTOMY
Before

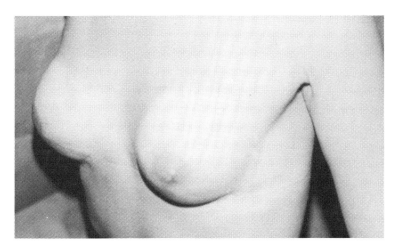

After

*Reconstruction of both
breasts*

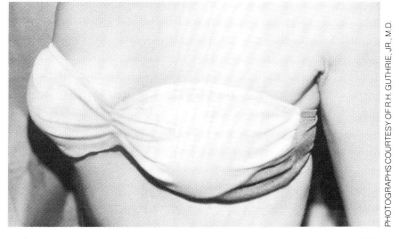

PHOTOGRAPHS COURTESY OF R.H. GUTHRIE, JR., M.D.

BREAST
REDUCTION
Before

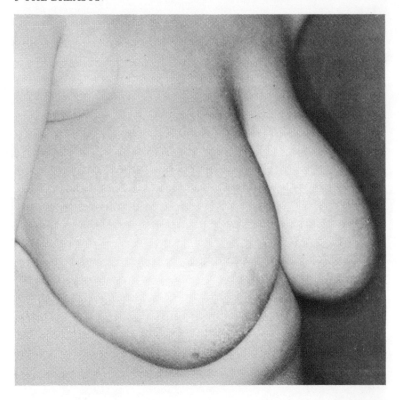

After

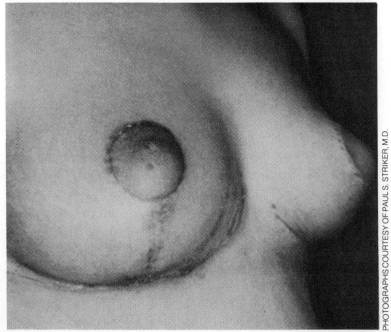

PHOTOGRAPHS COURTESY OF PAUL S. STRIKER, M.D.

218

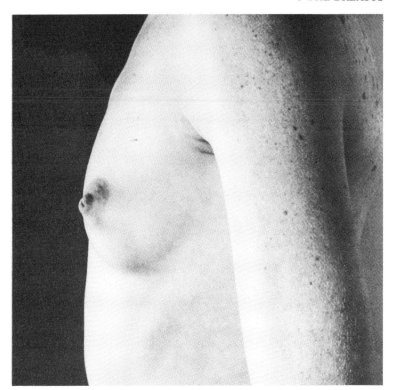

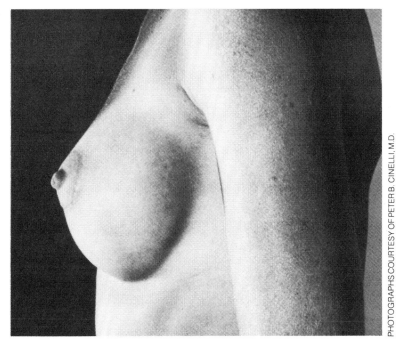

After

PHOTOGRAPHS COURTESY OF PETER B. CINELLI, M.D.

ASYMMETRICAL
BREASTS
Before

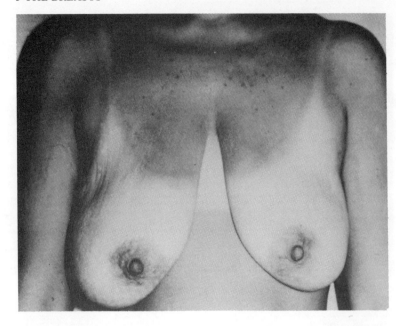

After
Reduction of left
breast; lifting of right
breast

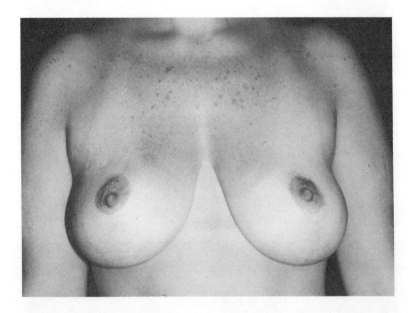

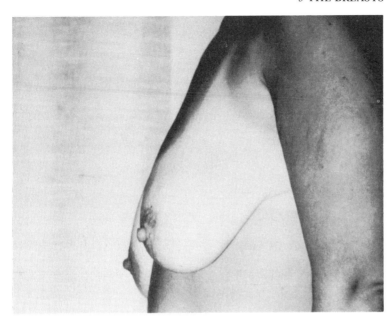

Side view
Before

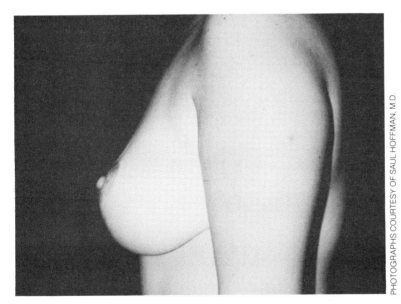

After

PHOTOGRAPHS COURTESY OF SAUL HOFFMAN, M.D.

10

Body Contouring:

Thigh, buttock, abdomen, arm, and hand

Before the 20th Century women modestly concealed their legs, hips, and torsos under flounces, bustles, and flowing gowns, exposing at most only a daring hint of décolletage. Although a tiny waist, molded by corsets and whalebone stays, was emphasized by elaborate Victorian styles, what lay below the waist was left to the imagination. The Victorian sensibility, plus the absence of electricity, no doubt prevented even a woman's husband from witnessing her without clothes, and if her shape below the waist was not ideal, it was not much in evidence either.

The 20th Century, however, inspired a new revelation of the female form. The first bathing suits were a scandal, although they covered as much of the body as possible. Later women began to wear short dresses, pants, gauzy synthetic fabrics, and finally bared all with miniskirts and bikinis. What fashions are now expected to reveal is not the voluptuous hourglass form of years gone by, but a narrow, athletic silhouette with little excess attached. Fashions are designed to show off slender legs and hips, and the woman who does not possess them naturally, or who has lost them through pregnancy, aging, or too little exercise combined with too much rich food, may find it difficult to wear the clothes suitable for the modern lifestyle and may feel embarrassed by the extra flesh. If she is overweight, a program of diet and exercise will bring her figure down to the desired shape, but there are some unaesthetic body formations which plastic surgeons call deformities that no amount of dieting, sit-ups, and leg lifts will banish.

After pregnancy, or a diet resulting in a large weight loss in a short time, a woman may find her once firm abdomen transformed into a gelatinous mass of loose skin. Pregnancy and surgery may produce unsightly stretch marks and abdominal scars. Loose flesh and scarring may make it embarrassing for her to wear a bikini, and a convex or flabby abdomen may make her outline in skirts, pants, and dresses less than ideal.

Some women also suffer from a deformity of the thighs

known as "riding breeches," which, as the name implies, are solid pads of bulging flesh on the outside of the legs, just below the hip. Riding breeches, often inherited, are stubbornly resistant to diet, exercise, or massage. The insides of the thighs and buttocks may sag with age or after sudden weight loss. For the same reasons, some women develop a deformity of the upper arms called "bat wings," or loose, dangling pendulums of flesh. All these figure problems sabotage a woman's silhouette, and sometimes her self-image and self-esteem. If she cannot accept her figure problem, or reduce it through diet and exercise, a woman can now find help from new procedures in plastic surgery that were designed to shape and contour specific areas of the body.

Body contouring operations were largely introduced in Brazil, and were further developed by American surgeons. The contouring procedures reduce and tighten flesh in places where it has outgrown the body structure on the abdomen, buttocks, and thighs. Contouring is also done on the upper arms and hands, although many surgeons are reluctant to operate on these areas. Generally known as the lipectomy, the contouring procedure is similar to altering a baggy dress. The surgeon estimates how much skin and tissue should be removed, makes an incision, removes the excess, sometimes redistributes tissues to mold the area into a more aesthetic shape, and sews a "seam," which brings the skin together again. The lipectomy, in short, is similar to a face lift on the abdomen, buttocks, and thighs. It sounds simple, but it is major surgery, done under general anesthesia in a hospital. Recovery time for all body contouring procedures ranges from six to eight weeks. Patients experience varying degrees of pain and inconvenience for at least two weeks after the operation.

Body contouring operations leave significant scars, as does all major surgery. How significant the scar is depends on the area where the procedure is done and the scarring capacity of each patient. The surgeon cannot predict the degree of scarring in advance, because everyone develops different kinds of scars, and different parts of the body scar differently as well. Scars on the torso, hands, and arms do not heal as well or as quickly as those on the face. Although the lipectomy has been developed to reduce the visibility of scars, all potential body contouring patients should understand they will be trading a silhouette for a scar. Patients unfortunate enough to be left with a really unsightly scar may have the results modified by another operation called "scar revision" in which a wide scar is made less prominent through an excision and resuturing procedure. At times a thickened scar is injected with cortisone in order to try to flatten it.

Because the surgery is major and scars result, body contouring operations are not for the mildly motivated or faint of heart, and potential patients should think twice before committing themselves. Surgeons try to impress on patients the gravity of the operation, and some are uneasy about performing it, especially on areas where scars are difficult to conceal. Said one eminent plastic surgeon:

We do these procedures but we are careful to select a highly motivated patient. We warn the patient about scars, but we can talk and talk and talk before the operation and there's still nothing like the result. If there's a bad scar afterwards, or the patient is disappointed with the result, it's psychologically bad for her and for the doctor. Scars mean different things to different people. They may be unattractive to the patient's husband, lover, or to herself. These operations, especially on the thighs, buttocks, upper arms, and hands, are for people who want to look good in clothes, not for people who want to expose their bodies.

Abdominoplasty

Surgeons do not consider the abdominal contouring procedure, or abdominoplasty, as disfiguring as other body contouring procedures because the scar can be concealed in the fold of the groin and just along the top line of pubic hair, thus allowing the patient to wear a bikini without embarrassment. Besides eliminating excess skin from the abdomen, the abdominoplasty can also correct damage to abdominal muscles and remove scars and stretch marks if they are located below the navel.

The operation called the abdominoplasty is a modern version of the abdominal lipectomy, which has been performed for medical reasons since 1910. The abdominoplasty is done to obtain cosmetic effects—shape and contour a sagging abdomen—whereas an abdominal lipectomy was only done for panniculus adiposus, or a fatty apron, a hanging, cone-shaped abdomen.

The fatty apron is not entirely fat, but a fold of loose, hanging skin which occurs when skin and adipose tissues in the abdomen lose resiliency, or when supporting muscle structures become weak and droop. Often caused when an obese person loses huge amounts of weight, the apron can also appear after pregnancy. A medical as well as an aesthetic problem, the apron causes the unwilling wearer extreme discomfort, feelings of heaviness, difficulties in moving, and sexual difficulties. The skin beneath the apron fold often becomes ulcerated, too. No amount of dieting affects the hanging fold of skin and it grows more pendulous and uncomfortable as the tissues involved are pulled earthward by gravity. Until recently, the apron was removed by making two incisions across the middle of the abdomen like a belt, or by making two intersecting incisions, one vertical and one horizon-

225

tal, and excising the extra skin and tissue in between. Both procedures produced a highly visible and unaesthetic scar, and now the apron is usually removed by the abdominoplasty technique. The more old-fashioned technique, however, involving a T-shaped or belt-shaped incision, is occasionally used for extreme cases of the fatty apron.

Usually the patient who requests an abdominoplasty for cosmetic reasons is a woman whose skin has lost the support of underlying tissues after dieting or pregnancy, leaving it stretched and loose. Since her problem is not overweight and since exercise strengthens muscles, not skin, no amount of dieting or exercise will alter the appearance of her abdomen. Often her skin is marred by stretch marks, which she also wants removed. Women who have had many pregnancies may suffer from diastasis recti, or the separation of the two straight muscles which run vertically on either side of the navel. The condition weakens and stretches the structure of the abdominal wall and may produce a convex abdomen or potbelly. Hernias, too, are sometimes an aftereffect of pregnancy. Both separated muscles and hernias are repaired during the contouring procedure. Some doctors feel the potbelly, which can be flattened with an abdominoplasty, can also be corrected by diligent exercise.

In men, who occasionally request abdominoplasty for cosmetic reasons, the surgical technique is slightly modified.

Abdominoplasty should never be mistaken for surgery to remove fat; its purpose is to tighten skin which has lost resiliency, repair muscles, and remove scars. The prognosis for patients with a tendency toward obesity is poor for major surgery of any kind. Overweight patients are more susceptible to infection, heal less quickly, and are inclined to high blood pressure and cardiac disease which makes general anesthesia less desirable.

The Consultation

What the doctor does during the abdominoplasty procedure is to try to move the skin from above the umbilicus, or navel, to the pubic region and to excise the skin that was originally situated below the navel. The best candidate for abdominoplasty is a woman who has stretch marks or scars she desires removed below the navel and the loose skin above it. The doctor carefully examines the skin of the patient's abdomen, checking as well for separated muscles and hernias. One doctor said:

We get a lot of requests for the abdominoplasty, but if there's not enough laxity in the skin so we can conceal the scar in the area of the groin, we don't do it.

As in all cosmetic procedures, the surgeon tries to determine the patient's motivation for the operation and avoids the patient who is not highly motivated or who thinks the operation will make a profound change in her life. The doctor then tries to impress upon the patient the seriousness of the operation and acquaint her with postoperative problems and scarring complications. He may show the patient before-and-after photographs of an abdominoplasty, warning her that results are different on everyone and no two people heal alike. The patient's general health is also carefully considered. The serious and lengthy surgical procedure can only be performed on healthy people; any systemic disease is a contraindication. If the patient is overweight, she will be asked to diet before the operation is considered.

Anne M., 26, was considered a good patient for abdominoplasty. Before her second pregnancy Anne weighed 115 pounds, although she is tall (5 feet 7 inches). During her second pregnancy she gained between 35 and 40 pounds and gave birth to a large child. She dieted and went down to her present weight of 123 pounds. She was dismayed, however, to find her once svelte abdomen marred with stretch marks and a loose fold of skin that remained impervious to exercise. Said Anne:

I didn't like the way I looked one bit and was embarrassed and unhappy about my "new" figure. I wouldn't have dreamed of trying to wear even a one-piece bathing suit. I also had an umbilical hernia which needed to be repaired. I think the prospect of the operation frightened my husband and I had to coax him before he would agree to it.

The abdominoplasty successfully trims the silhouette and flattens and firms a sagging or convex abdomen. Since most of the fatty tissue in the belly is located below the navel, and the skin above the navel that is moved down to replace it has less fatty tissue, the operation can succeed in eliminating fat, although that is not its major purpose. Many surgeons automatically tighten the rectus muscles along the abdomen with sutures, whether they are separated or not, which makes the waistline appear more slender. Tightening the muscles surgically is equivalent to tightening them through exercise. The patient should remember, however, that her abdomen is being slenderized, not totally transformed; she should not expect to end up with the same figure she had at 16, only a slightly better one than she had before the operation.

The stretch marks above the navel will not be eliminated by the procedure, but they will be smoothed out. If the stretch marks and loose skin were caused by pregnancy, they may recur if the patient becomes pregnant again.

What to Expect from an Abdominoplasty

227

The patient should also remember that there is a long recovery period for abdominoplasty, and she will not be able to enjoy her new silhouette immediately after leaving the hospital. Said Anne M:

I was terribly disappointed by the results in the beginning. With my belly swollen from surgery and what looked like huge scars, I wondered what in the world I'd been thinking of when I decided to have the operation. But now, 11 months later, I'm glad. My belly is flat. The scars have faded and are now the same color as the rest of my skin. They seem to have gotten smaller. I still have some stretch marks but they're completely smooth. We were in Puerto Rico a short time ago and I wore a bikini, just as I used to.

Preoperative Procedures

The patient should not take aspirin or medication containing aspirin for two weeks prior to surgery. She shaves the pubic area herself a few days before she enters the hospital, or it is shaved on the operating table so the doctor can easily discern the top of the pubic hairline. Sometimes patients are advised to bathe with a disinfectant soap two weeks prior to surgery to prevent infection; however, one disinfectant bath the day before entering the hospital may be deemed sufficient. Phenobarbital may be given the night before surgery and an intramuscular injection one hour before surgery. The doctor visits the patient before the operation and marks the incision line on her abdomen with a special pen while she is standing. He estimates the amount of skin he will excise, hoping that he can remove the entire area below the navel region, but final decision on the amount to be excised is made during surgery. One doctor said:

I ask the patient to bring a bikini to the hospital—not a skimpy one but a bikini—so I will be able to plan the incision inside the bikini line.

The doctor also measures the exact location of the umbilicus so it will not be pulled out of position during the stretching and suturing of the skin.

The Surgical Procedure for Abdominoplasty

The operation is done under general anesthesia. The patient is placed in a jackknife position that puts the abdomen in a relaxed position, making it easier for the doctor to close the incision without tension on the suture line. The surgeon makes his first incision in the shape of a W along the lines he has drawn on the patient before the operation. The center point of the W is located on the midline of the abdomen, just above the top line of pubic hair, and the "legs" of the W extend along the fold of the groin. The final scar will appear along the same lines. This W incision

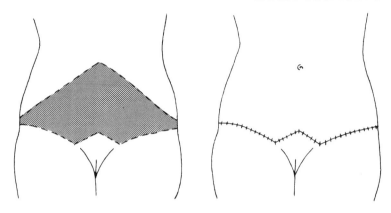

Abdominoplasty corrects a sagging abdomen. The shaded portion indicates the area of skin to be excised. Skin above the navel is stretched down to replace the flabby, striated skin below. The final sutures are not apparent when the patient wears a bikini.

was designed to place a minimal scar in the concealing fold of the groin and the upper line of the pubic hair. Other surgical techniques are sometimes employed.

After the incision has been made, the surgeon undermines the skin, or lifts it from the tissue beneath, all the way up to the rib cage, creating a flap. He stretches the loose skin downwards and pulls it inwards; as he excises the excess tissue, he makes a second incision. In order to maintain the original position of the umbilicus, the surgeon cuts around it, leaving it on an island connected to its blood supply, then creates a new opening for it in the skin which is moved down over it. In other words, the navel doesn't move but is surrounded by new skin. Once situated in its new opening, the navel is sutured into place. In a bikini the faint scar around the umbilicus should be the only telltale sign of an abdominoplasty. During the operation the doctor repairs the separated abdominal muscles, or slims the waistline, by tightening them with a heavy suture thread.

The most demanding part of the procedure occurs when the surgeon decides how much skin to excise and closes the wound. Some doctors use an instrument called a flap demarcator—a long clamp which enables him to measure accurately and mark off the amount to be cut. If the surgeon stretches the skin too tightly over the abdomen, closing it under too much tension, complications may result; on the other hand, if he does not excise enough excess skin, the cosmetic effect may be less than expected. The entire procedure takes from three to five hours.

Postoperative
Procedure

The postoperative course varies with doctors and patients. Usually the patient remains in the hospital about five days. She must lie on her back with her legs bent and slightly elevated. Suction drains are placed under the skin during the operation, which help it adhere to its new location on the muscle tissue and prevent fluid from accumulating under the flap. The drains remain for three to five days. The abdomen is dressed with a nonadherent gauze next to the skin and large gauze pads. Since complications like pneumonia may occur if patients do not move soon enough after surgery, some doctors ask the patient to dangle her legs from the bed on the first day after the operation. By the second day the patient begins to walk bent over.

Once home from the hospital the patient is not allowed to stand up straight or sit down for about two weeks and she would find it painful if she did. Coughing, sneezing, and laughing, which utilize stomach muscles, may also be painful. Some of the sutures are removed after a week and by the third week all of them are out. A soft, elastic girdle is generally recommended for four to six weeks. Patients see the doctor several times for the first month, with longer intervals between succeeding visits. Anne M. described her postoperative experience:

I can't say it was too bad an ordeal. I was in the hospital for four days, but out of bed and walking around the day after surgery—slightly bent over but otherwise not in pain. I stayed bent over for about three weeks before I could straighten up. Straightening up was very uncomfortable and it was impossible to stretch out in bed, too. I kept a pillow under my knees with my legs bent—that put less strain on the incision. I rested a great deal for the first week at home, but after that I was able to do things for myself. It was six weeks before I felt completely normal. My abdomen was swollen for four weeks. By the seventh week after the operation I was playing tennis and completely myself.

Complications

When the abdominoplasty is done by a competent surgeon, complications are uncommon. However, if the skin is stretched too tightly across the abdomen as a result of an overenthusiastic excision, fluid may accumulate under the skin flap or the blood supply to the skin can be damaged and an area of the skin can die. This rarely occurs but when it does, skin may have to be grafted in the area of skin loss. Fluid accumulation may also occur from too much activity after surgery. Blood clots can form if the patient's blood pressure rises after the operation. Infection, too, is a possibility.

Bad scarring is possible if the incision is not closed under the proper tension. The type of scar that develops along the incision line will not be fully apparent for about one year. Patients should

230

reserve judgment about the final result until that time has elapsed. Occasionally blood transfusions are necessary.

The surgeon's fee for abdominoplasty ranges from $1,500 to $5,000. The average fee is about $2,500. Hospital costs and the anesthesiologist's fee are not included. Sometimes medical insurance will cover the operation if the patient suffers from separated muscles, hernias, or an abdomen badly scarred from previous surgery.

Fees

Some women suffer from a deformity of the thighs known as trochanteric lipodystrophy, or "riding breeches." These recalcitrant pads of flesh on the outside of the thighs just below the hip afflict only women, whose inclination to store fat below the waist is considered a secondary sex characteristic. Although heavyset women are more disposed to riding breeches, slender women may be burdened with them too. The cause of riding breeches is not known. The condition cannot be attributed to glandular dysfunction or obesity. Doctors suspect a hereditary trait.

The Thigh and Buttock Lift

In France these diet-resistant and exercise-resistant pads of flesh are called cellulite, or orange skin, because of their tough, dimpled appearance. The French believe that massage, more than diet or exercise regimens, can help dissolve them. In America, however, the Food and Drug Administration has banned the word cellulite from advertising campaigns, because research has proved there is no biological difference between the fat cells in these stubborn areas and those in ordinary fat.

The woman who has dieted down to minimum weight, however, and finds her riding breeches unbudged, does not feel the unaesthetic pads to be ordinary fat. Although no health problems are associated with riding breeches, they create a disconcerting bulge in sports clothes or narrow skirts and may force a woman to purchase clothing a size larger than the rest of her body needs. Women with riding breeches often can't fit into slacks (except, of course, for jodhpurs) or feel embarrassed to be seen in them. Said Lisa, who is a petite 5 feet 1 inch tall, age 30 journalist:

I was always a small, slim girl, but when I became 12, fat pads developed on the sides of my hips. My thighs had always been heavy, but the addition of lumps on the sides added a new, unwelcome dimension. I dieted and exercised, but nothing diminished them. I suppose it doesn't sound like the worst tragedy in the world, but to a self-conscious adolescent, these pads were a serious disfigurement. It was impossible for me to wear pants. I couldn't ski because you can't ski very well in skirts. When everyone went to the picnic in jeans and a T-shirt, there I was in a full or

231

A-line skirt. I felt different and self-conscious and, finally, depressed. I used to fantasize about waking up one morning with a body shaped like everyone else's.

Other women are unhappy to find their inner thighs sagging from age or from sudden weight loss; buttocks can succumb to the same fate. The loose tissue in these areas is pulled downward by gravity and, like riding breeches, may make a woman's body image less appealing than she would like.

Riding breeches can now be removed. The same incision that eliminates them can be adapted to lift sagging buttocks and inner thighs. Surgeons used to perform a lift on the inner thigh alone, but this technique involved making a vertical incision down the length of the thigh and left an unsightly scar. The thigh and buttock lift, as the operation is called, is more complicated to perform than abdominoplasty and leaves part of the resulting scar in a visible area above the hip bone. For this reason it is avoided by some plastic surgeons.

What to Expect from a Thigh and Buttock Lift

Fat that is surgically removed does not tend to recur. Consequently the riding breeches operation will probably rid the patient of unwanted fat pads forever. Actually, fat is not usually excised during the procedure, but readjusted and pulled up toward the buttock, giving the leg a smoother contour. Patients should keep in mind, however, that though the bulging pads will be reduced, the entire thigh area will not appear slimmer after the operation; only the contour, not the general structure or weight of the leg, will be changed.

If the doctor extends the same incision he makes to eliminate riding breeches around to the front of the thigh, the lax skin on the inner thigh can be tightened. Gravity, however, will probably pull the skin of the thigh back down. One surgeon said: "Gravity is against us on the inner thigh. The patient would need a full-time policeman to hold the tissues up permanently." The incision to eliminate riding breeches also eliminates the lower third of the buttock, which makes it appear smaller. Since sagging buttock skin accumulates in the lower part of the buttock, it too will be removed. Aging and the pull of gravity may cause the buttock to sag again, however. The scar from the procedure is hidden in the buttock fold and the crease of the groin in front. Part of it extends up to the hipbone area, just below the bikini line. The scar will take a year to mature.

Consultation with a Physician

The patient is acquainted with the serious nature of the operation and warned about the resulting scars. Like the abdominoplasty patient, she may be shown before-and-after photographs

232

of the procedure and told that all results are not the same. The patient should be highly motivated and must understand that the purpose of the operation is to improve her appearance in clothes. She should not be in poor health or overweight.

The preoperative procedures are the same as for the abdominoplasty, except the pubic region is not shaved. The doctor visits the patient before the operation, estimates how much skin and tissue will be removed during the procedure, and draws incision lines while she is standing.

Preoperative Procedures

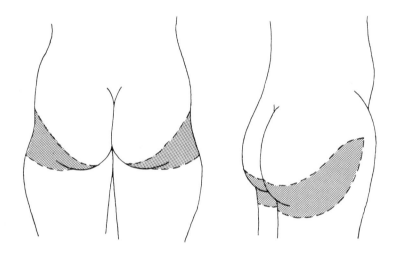

Thigh and buttock lift corrects "riding breeches." Wing-shaped shaded portions indicate the areas of skin and tissue to be removed.

The operation is usually done in a hospital under general anesthesia. The anesthetized patient is placed on her abdomen on the operating table. This process can be lengthy because the doctor must make sure that she is in exactly the right position and that all her extremities are resting on pads; otherwise, pressure sores and possibly paralysis might occur.

The Surgical Procedure for Thigh and Buttock Lift

To lift the thigh and buttock the doctor makes two incisions producing a wing-shaped flap, which begins in the area just below the final third of the buttock and ends below the buttock's crease. This flap will be excised, and the skin of the thigh pulled up to meet the edge of the remaining skin of the buttock, creating a tighter, smoother contour to the thigh. The incision line extends the full length of the buttock, then curves around and up toward the hip bone. The undermined area, or flap, includes the area where riding breeches are located. How far up the hip the scar extends depends on the degree of lift that is necessary. Basically, the surgeon readjusts the fatty tissue that composes the riding breeches, molding it and pulling it up toward the buttock, so it no longer creates a protruberant lump. Sometimes excess fatty tissue is removed, although the removal of fat may endanger the blood supply and is avoided. The surgeon also avoids undermining skin he does not plan to excise, to avoid depressions in the thigh when the operation is complete.

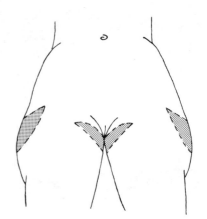

For an inner thigh lift, the incision for correcting riding breeches is carried to the inner side of the thighs.

If the inner thigh is to be lifted too, the wing-shaped incision is continued around to the front of the patient's body; the sagging skin is pulled up and the excess is removed. Since a lower third of the patient's buttock falls within the two incision lines, its natural fold will be excised, eliminating an unsightly depression in some patients. The tissue of the buttock, too, can be molded into a more aesthetic shape during the procedure. The entire operation, it should be remembered, was designed to remove riding breeches, but can be tailored to contour the buttocks and lift the inner thigh. Few women, however, request the operation to contour the inner thigh or buttock alone.

The surgeon closes the two edges of skin with sutures, effectively creating a new buttock crease, where the final suture line and final scar will be placed. "If we were to suture the skin along the old buttock crease, gravity would soon pull the scar downward toward the thigh," said one surgeon. Since scars in areas of tension (created here by sitting) tend to widen, the doctor tries to keep the scar small to begin with by suturing the area with subcutaneous suture lines, or by weaving the stitches beneath the skin and letting the ends of the thread emerge on either end of

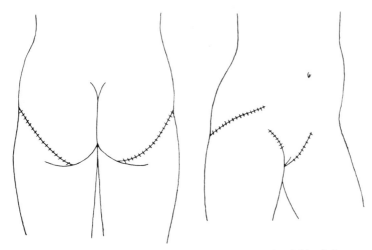

The final sutures of a thigh and buttock lift follow the fold of the buttock and extend almost to the hipbone.

the suture line. Other complex surgical procedures are done to ensure the smallest possible scar. The entire operation takes three and a half hours, or longer if the inner thighs are lifted too.

As in abdominoplasty, it is important that the surgeon not excise too much skin and that he close the wound with just the proper degree of tension. If he excises too much skin, tissue complications occur; if he doesn't excise enough, the cosmetic effect will not be satisfactory. One patient, who experienced considerable discomfort after the operation, had unfortunately engaged an excellent surgeon who was not, however, experienced in the riding breeches procedure. She said:

To my disappointment the operation had accomplished nothing. The bulges were slightly, slightly reduced but the same problem essentially remained. Six months later I returned to the doctor and he offered to repeat the operation without charge. He had improved his technique and this time the result was better, but not perfect. If I gain the slightest bit of weight there's a depression at the sides of my thighs where the incision was made. The scars are most evident—they go under the buttocks and up the sides of the hips, but I can wear a modified bikini, pants and jeans, and slim straight skirts. In clothes I have a reasonably normal body and feel I can lead a normal life. In spite of the disappointments and problems of the two operations, I'm glad I did it.

The patient must remain in the hospital for five to seven days after the operation. Suction drains are inserted in the buttock area. She lies on her back with her hips flexed in order to relieve

Postoperative Procedure

235

tension on the suture line. In a day or two the patient is asked to begin walking. Too much bed rest may result in lung complications or thrombophlebitis. The suture lines are bandaged with a gauze dressing. Sutures are removed 8 to 14 days after surgery. Once at home, the patient may only walk or recline. She may not sit for two or three weeks, because sitting places tension on the suture line. It is also very painful. Said Lisa F. of her postoperative experience:

I was in the hospital for ten days (longer than usual). The pain was intense. I could not sit or go to the bathroom. I had to lie on my stomach for the first few days. There were rubber drains under the buttocks. The first six weeks were an ordeal of intense pain. I was able to return to work eight weeks after the operation. I still had some discomfort, but no real pain.

Possible
Complications

Possible complications for the thigh and buttock lift include fluid accumulation under the flap, and skin loss, which can occur if the suture line is closed under too much tension. Grave scarring may also occur if the suture line is closed under tension, and the patient's vagina or anus may be stretched open. Blood clots and loss of blood (requiring transfusion) may occur during surgery. Infections are also possible. Lymphedema, or swelling of the legs, may also occur. If the operation is competently performed, complications are rare.

Fees

The surgeon's fee for a thigh and buttock lift ranges from $1,500 to $5,000. The average fee is $2,500. The fee is the same whether the inner thigh is lifted or not, and the same if only the inner thigh or buttock is lifted. Hospital costs and the anesthesiologist's fee are extra. Insurance will not cover any of the expenses since, unlike abdominoplasty, there are no medical indications for the operation.

Upper Arm
Lipectomy

Women develop bat-wing deformity or upper arm lipodystrophy from sudden weight loss or aging. The loose skin that hangs down from the arm is pulled further downward by gravity and may make the arm appear unaesthetic even in sleeves. Excision of extra tissue in the upper arm region is seldom done by plastic surgeons in this country, however, because it leaves scars that do not mature well. Some surgeons have tried to minimize the visibility of the scar by creating a sinuous incision line instead of a straight vertical incision along the inside of the arm. Other surgeons pull the lax skin up toward the armpit and excise it there. In the majority of cases, the operation leaves disfiguring scars. Said one surgeon:

236

I did a few of these operations in residency and the scars were ghastly.
Some parts of the body don't heal well and I think the upper arm is one of
them. I won't do the operation at all now.

As hands begin to age the skin on the back of the hand may become loose and wrinkled, disfigured by brown age spots and protruding veins. Lipectomy of the hand, called hand rhytido-plasty, can be performed by pulling the wrinkled and sagging skin tight across the back of the hand and excising the excess by making an incision that runs from just below the wrist to the beginning of the little finger. Again, most surgeons do not perform this operation because of the unsightly nature of the final scar. Dermabrasion is not recommended to remove brown age spots for the same reason—the skin of the hand is thin and delicate and scars easily. Small amounts of silicone, however, can be injected between the protruding veins to even out the surface of the skin.

Cosmetic Procedures for the Hand

Men and women suffering from arthritis may have hands that are seriously disfigured and crippled. A recent development in plastic surgery involves replacing the natural joints in arthritic hands with artificial joints made out of silicone rubber. The new joints give arthritis sufferers more mobility in their hands and enable them to do simple tasks that had been impossible. They improve the appearance of the hands vastly. During a complex procedure the doctor removes the diseased bones and inserts the new joints into one end of the bone and down through the canal of the other. Tendons are repaired to strengthen the fingers as well. After surgery a trained therapist works with the patients to help them regain hand movements.

**THIGH AND
BUTTOCK LIFT**

Before

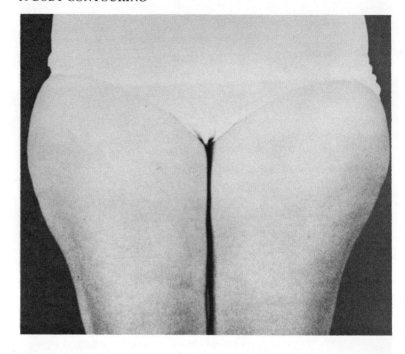

After

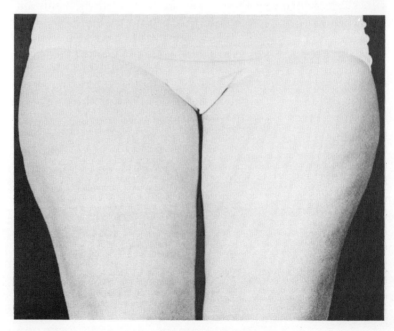

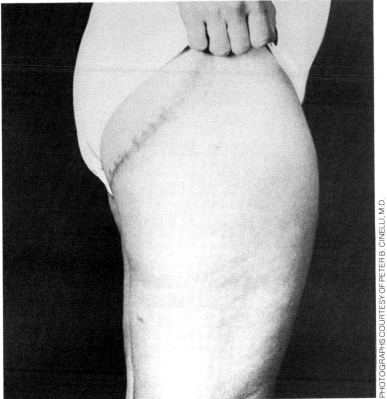

Side view showing scars six months postoperatively

PHOTOGRAPHS COURTESY OF PETER B. CINELLI, M.D.

ABDOMINO-
PLASTY
Before

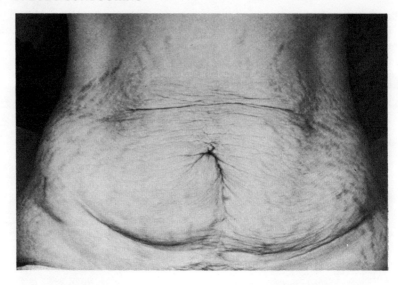

After

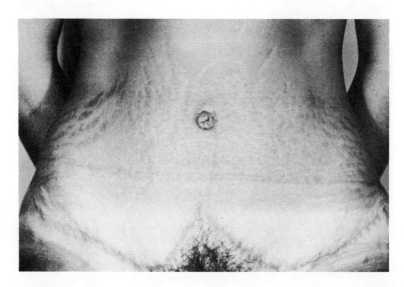

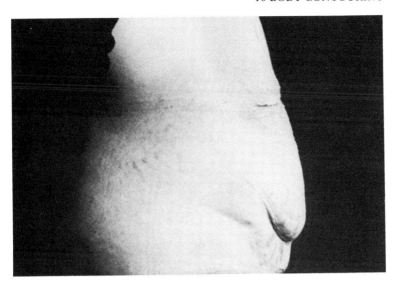

Side view
Before

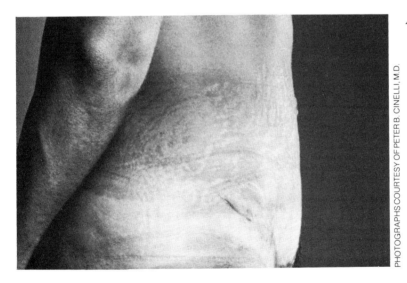

After

PHOTOGRAPHS COURTESY OF PETER B. CINELLI, M.D.

241

ABDOMINOPLASTY
Before

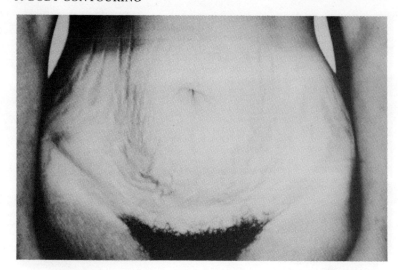

After

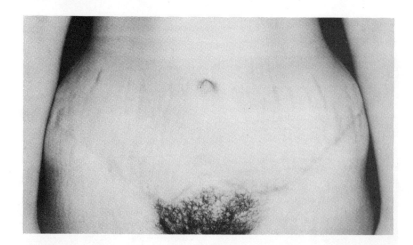

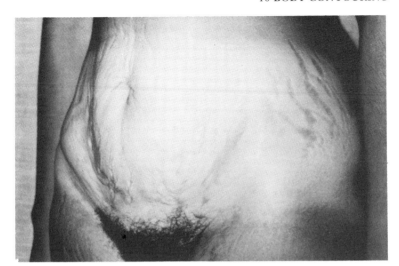

Three-quarter view before

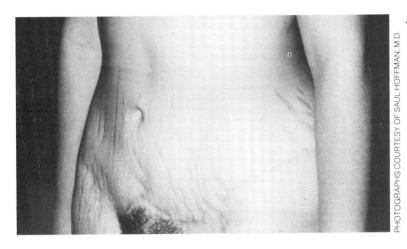

After

PHOTOGRAPHS COURTESY OF SAUL HOFFMAN, M.D.

ABDOMINOPLASTY
FATTY APRON
Before

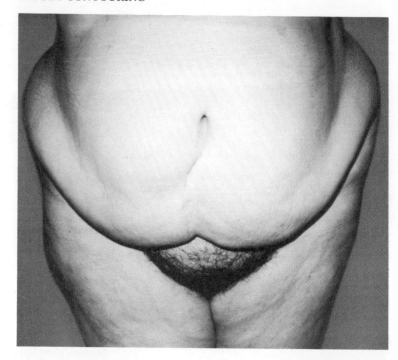

After

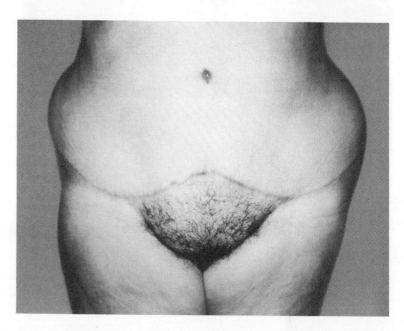

244

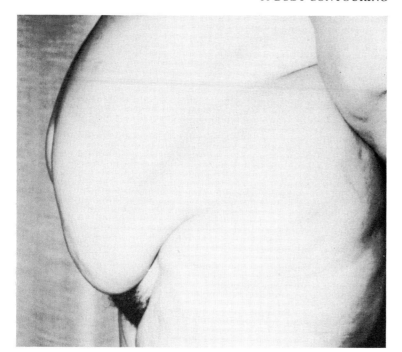

Side view
Before

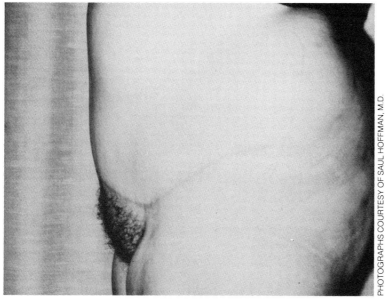

After

PHOTOGRAPHS COURTESY OF SAUL HOFFMAN, M.D.

Glossary

adipose Fatty.

Adrenalin Trade name for a drug (epinephrine) used to raise blood pressure and slow bleeding.

ala Any winglike process; refers particularly to the outer portion of each nostril, which consists of skin and cartilage.

analgesic A painkiller that does not induce loss of consciousness.

antihelix The curved ridge of the external ear just below the helix.

areola The pigmented circular area around the nipple of the breast.

asepsis Maintenance of sterility; exclusion of micro-organisms.

auricle The external ear.

axilla The armpit.

bite Relative position of upper and lower teeth.

blepharoplasty Plastic surgery of the eyelids.

canthus The corner on either side of the eyes where the upper and lower lids meet.

capillaries Tiny blood vessels.

carcinogenic Having the ability to induce cancer.

carcinoma A malignant growth (cancer).

cartilage A firm, elastic, translucent substance comprising part of the skeleton; gristle.

cheiloplasty Plastic surgery of the lips.

chemosurgery Application of chemical substances to the skin to produce an intense burn that induces exfoliation, or peeling.

clavicle The collarbone.

collagen The main supportive protein of skin, tendon, bone, cartilage, and connective tissue.

columella The fleshy column below the tip of the nose.

congenital A condition existing at birth.

conjunctiva The mucous membrane lining the eyelids and covering a portion of the eyeball.

cutaneous Pertaining to the skin.

dermabrasion Mechanical abrasion (sanding) of the skin to remove the top layers.

dermatitis Inflammation of the skin.

dermis The layer of skin that is below the epidermis (top layer).

ectropion A turning outward, especially of the lower eyelids.

edema Swelling of soft tissues due to excessive accumulation of fluid.

epidermis The outer layer of the skin.

fascia A layer of thick fibrous tissue sheathing the muscles.

flap A partially detached portion of skin and tissue carrying its own blood supply.

glabella The area between the eyebrows.

graft The moving of tissue from one part of the body to another.

helix The rounded rim of the external ear.

hematoma An abnormal collection of blood in the tissues, resulting from injury or surgery.

hemostasis The control of bleeding.

hyper- A prefix meaning excessive, over, above.

hypertrophy Enlargement or overgrowth.

hypo- A prefix meaning beneath, under, below.

keloid The abnormal thickening of a scar caused by overgrowth of scar tissue.

keratosis Localized, thickened, scaly area of the skin.

labial Pertaining to the lips.

lipectomy Excision of fatty tissue.

malocclusion Abnormal relationship between upper and lower teeth.

mammaplasty Plastic surgery of the breast.

mandible The lower jawbone.

mastectomy Surgical removal of the breast.

maxilla The upper jawbone.

melanin The dark pigment in the skin and hair.

mentoplasty Plastic surgery of the chin.

mucosa Mucous membrane.

nasolabial fold Fold running from the side of the nose to the upper lip.

obesity Accumulation of fat in the body.

orbit Bony cavity of the skull that contains the eye.

osteotomy Excision of bone or portion of it.

otoplasty Plastic surgery of the ear.

prognathia Overdevelopment of the lower jaw with malocclusion.

prosthesis An artificial substitute for a missing part of the body.

ptosis Drooping or abnormal lowering of an organ or tissue of the body. (adj.: ptotic)

pulmonary Relating to the lungs.

rhinoplasty Plastic surgery of the nose.

rhytidoplasty Plastic surgery to remove facial sags and folds; a face lift.

sebaceous Pertaining to microscopic glands in the skin that secrete a waxy substance known as sebum.

septum A partition between two spaces or cavities, such as the nasal septum.

striae Streaks or stripes commonly known as "stretch marks," due to rupture of elastic fibers of the skin.

submental Under the chin.

suture A thread used for surgical sewing or (verb) to close a wound by stitching skin edges together.

telangiectasis Dilation of groups of capillaries.

umbilicus The navel or belly button.

vermilion The red mucosa of the lips.

Index